Born for Life: A Midwife's Story

Born for Life: A Midwife's Story by Julie Watson.
Published by Cherry Hinton Limited.
Copyright © 2015 Cherry Hinton Limited.
The author can be contacted at: cherryhintonlimited@gmail.com

Disclaimer: This book is a work of non-fiction by the author. Some names have been changed to protect the privacy of the individuals involved. Any websites listed were current at the time of printing.

Printed in New Zealand by PublishMe Self Publishing.
www.publishme.co.nz

ISBN: 978-0-473-29963-7

This title is also available in eBook format.
Epub ISBN: 978-0-473-29964-4
Mobi ISBN: 978-0-473-29965-1
iBook ISBN: 978-0-473-29966-8

Born for Life

A Midwife's Story

A life story written by
Julie Watson

Contents

Prologue

"Next push and we will have the baby," he said. The baby's head seemed to be turned to the side now and with the next contraction I saw the doctor pull the baby down as the shoulders were released and the body slid out.

"Nurse, give that injection," I was told by Sister while the doctor got a tube and put it down the baby's throat.

"Whaa, whaa, whaa," the baby was crying lustily and became pink from a slightly blue colour. I looked down at the crying baby who lay on the draw sheet, wet and naked, arms and legs moving wildly.

'Wow! My first baby. How amazing!' I thought.

Shaking slightly, I took the syringe, put the needle into the leg where Sister had told me to and pushed the fluid inside. Sister put a plastic clamp on the umbilical cord near the baby and she put another large metal clamp about two inches from the plastic clamp. Then, taking some scissors from the trolley, she cut the umbilical cord between the two.

"You have a baby boy, Emma," Doctor Symes said as he took the clamped end of the cord.

The baby was now unattached. Sister dried him with a towel and, wrapping the baby up, handed it to its relieved mother, who just gazed down at her baby, beaming and smiling. She looked a picture of happiness and contentment as she held her newborn in her arms. Such a stark contrast to what had been just a few short minutes ago.

I didn't see the afterbirth come out, but the next time I looked on the trolley, a metal kidney dish with a soft, bloody, spongy object was in it. The dish was barely big enough, as it lapped over the edge.

Next thing I knew, Sister was taking the bottom part of the bed apart and preparing for the doctor to do the suturing.

"Nurse, help me with these poles will you?" Sister brought the tall stainless steel poles, which were curved at one end with straps hanging from them, over from the corner of the room. She started showing me how to put them in at the end of the bed so that we could put Mrs Little's legs up and secure them with the straps. Her legs were now wide apart and her feet were secured on top of the poles ready for Doctor Symes to suture the perineum.

I was excited and elated at seeing my first baby being born and felt so privileged to have such an amazing job. I was on a high and enthusiastically buzzed around doing all that needed to be done.

When the suturing was finished, we took Mrs Little's legs down and put the bed back together. Sister and I sponged Mrs Little down with warm water, soap and a flannel and then swabbed her perineum – the area between the anus and the opening of the vagina – with Savlon, put on a clean pad, then a tight abdominal binder. The binder was pinned all the way down, from just below her breast to the material pad, and secured at the back by another safety pin. While we did this, Doctor Symes checked the baby over before writing in the notes and heading off.

We wheeled Mrs Little back into the labour room to be reunited with her husband. With her new son in her arms, she brought him to her breast and gave him his first feed. I made a cup of tea for Mrs Little and her husband, as well as for Sister and myself. Sister Foster took her cup of tea and all the paperwork into the office while I quickly gulped down mine and started the clean up. The theatre had to be cleaned and put back together in readiness for the next delivery. The bowls and instruments needed to be cleaned and put in a bundle to be sterilized.

When all was finished, Sister and I wheeled the new mother on her bed down the ward to the postnatal room, where she would be staying for the next week or so.

This was to be the first of many more labours and births, and the first of many women I would be with during childbirth. It was the start of my love for being with women, helping them through their pain and supporting them as they gave birth to their precious babies. It was such a rewarding feeling seeing all the pain turn into joy and gratitude when the baby was finally born. To see a woman fall in love instantly with the baby that she had given birth to, and forget all the pain she had gone through, seemed to me a miracle.

Born for Life

The Beginning

WHEN DID THE DREAM START? When did the journey begin? My grandmother gave me a small Ladybird book as part of my birthday present when I was ten years old. Reading the life of Florence Nightingale, I decided that being a nurse was what I wanted to do when I grew up. Imagining that, like Florence, I would be able to heal the sick and bring hope to people with my care and compassion. I imagined tending the sick and dying in a war zone in some far off land.

I thought a lot in my childhood about what I would do in life. Along with wanting to become a nurse, I also wanted to be a circus performer, an air hostess, an Olympic swimmer and even an actress. One by one though, my dreams would come crashing down. In my circus phase, I put a hole through the bedroom wall doing somersaults off the bed. Dad was not impressed and I was severely reprimanded. My circus career ended before it began. In my swimming phase, I can remember nearly drowning at least a couple of times. Dad rescued me from the river at a Lions' Christmas picnic. I was walking to the other side of the river with a friend, hand in hand. My friend, who I was walking with, was a lot taller than I was. So as we walked, I was going deeper under the water. Fortunately,

Dad spotted us before my head completely disappeared. Then, again, on holiday in Rotorua, I jumped into the deep end of the swimming pool, still unable to swim. I remember all the hands coming down to grab me out of the pool as I kept coming up to the surface and then going down into the water again. I copped another scolding from Dad who was usually quiet, loving and sedate. He seemed rather stressed as he pulled me from the water, telling me to never jump in a pool again without finding out which was the deep end.

The nursing dream seemed to be the only one where I didn't have my bubble burst and where no discouragement came to destroy it. So I carried my dream of becoming a nurse from the time I read the book until I wanted to leave school. My mother decided that working at the local hospital as a nurse aide was good enough and didn't see any need for me to go away and do formal training.

She knew the matron of the local hospital and, while talking to her one day in town, my mother asked her if there was a vacancy for me as a nurse aide at the hospital. I had finished school at the end of the fifth form because I was bored and impatient to run my own life.

I had been rebellious in the fourth form and had never really regained my love of school. As my grades had dropped, I struggled to keep up. Amazing how a year of mucking about, having some fun and not applying oneself, puts you back so much that it's virtually impossible to regain the ground lost. So leaving school seemed to be the best option and jobs were easy to find in 1970. My first job was at the local shoe shop for six months, before I got the call from the matron to start work at Pahiatua Hospital.

This is what I had dreamed of. Also, as I was earning $12.50 a week at the shoe shop and I was going to be earning $52 a fortnight at the hospital, it seemed too good an opportunity to miss. A doubling in wages overnight seemed like a small fortune, so there was no doubt about taking the offer.

I had a boyfriend, Barry, whom I had been going out with since I was fifteen years old. He didn't want me to leave town to do formal nursing training and especially not to Palmerston North, which was 40 minutes away. There were rumours of girls sneaking out at night from the nurses' home there and boys being sneaked into the nurses' quarters, where drinking and sex were rumoured to be rife.

Heck no, Barry didn't want to risk losing me to that and at the moment I was satisfied and happy. At least I was going to be a nurse, not a trained one, but a nurse nevertheless.

As I walked up the driveway, I admired the beautiful rose gardens that were uniformly placed around and the perfectly manicured lawn with trees lining the hospital boundary. Surrounding the buildings were masses of colour from the flower beds, with edges trimmed and not a weed in sight. The driveway curved around, going from the main hospital and offices to the maternity annexe at the far end of the hospital grounds

The main part of the hospital was made of red brick, large and square in shape. There was a long corridor going from the main hospital to the maternity annexe. It was painted cream with rough caste plaster up to the windows, then plain plaster above that was also painted cream with a green board separating the two. The roof of the hospital was covered with red corrugated iron.

Nervousness and apprehension stopped me from fully appreciating the beauty and tranquillity of the hospital grounds as I made my way to the large front door.

My heart pounding, I waited by the main office for Mrs Sinclair to call me in for the fitting of my uniform. Finally, she came out of a side door in the corridor and called me into the little sewing room. She had a tape measure in hand to measure the length of my uniform, which had to be around knee length and not too tight around the bust. The uniform was a white, short-sleeved dress that was slightly stiff and buttoned all the way up the front. There were buttonholes on both sides of the uniform.

Down one side of the front, the buttons went through the buttonholes and were secured at the back by a metal clip. The buttons were round and white with a metal eyelet at the back. A metal clip was put through the eyelet at the back to secure it in place. These buttons were taken off after each shift and the uniform put into the laundry. The nurse aides had cardboard hats that came flat and we had to fold them into shape and then clip them onto our hair. The trained nurses, or sisters, and the matron all had fabric hats.

"You will have to buy some white stockings and white shoes and you will need a red cardigan for when it gets cold," Mrs Sinclair said.

"Your uniforms and cape will be in a locker in maternity when you start. I'll have them all named for you. The locker will have your name on it and a key in the lock."

The nurse aides had blue capes lined with red and the trained nurses had red capes lined with blue. I must say, I felt a sense of pride as I tried the cape on. It had a thick, wide collar and there were two straps that came down on either side that crossed over in front and buttoned at the back. The capes were made of a thick, woollen material and felt very warm. They were not to be worn while tending to patients but could be worn at other times and, like the uniform, were not to be worn home.

After I had finished being measured up, Mrs Sinclair showed me to a seat where I was to wait for Mrs Brunton, the matron, who wanted to see me and give me a tour of the hospital.

I had never met Mrs Brunton before and my nervousness worsened while waiting outside the door of her office. There was no mistaking who she was when the door eventually opened and an older, greyhaired lady came over to greet me.

"Hello, you must be Julie. Mrs Sinclair tells me she has finished measuring you up for your uniforms. She'll have them ready for you by the time you start next Monday. Now come with me and I'll take you to meet Sister Foster. She is expecting us over in maternity. That's where you will come when you start. I am sure you will enjoy working at the hospital and maternity is such a nice place to work."

I stood up and all I could say was, "Yes. Thank you."

I was intimidated and in awe of this woman who looked a lot older than my mother and had an air of grace and authority about her. She was dressed in a white uniform similar to the one I had tried on, but with long sleeves that were cuffed at the wrists. She looked almost regal, as she also wore a white veil that flowed down past her shoulders. The veil was made of a fine material and the hat itself was stiff and clipped to her grey, wavy hair. She looked like a nun, but dressed in white not black.

I had never met anyone with the sense of presence that she had. I spoke quietly when she spoke to me, nodded in the appropriate places and felt I had to almost bow in her presence. Her smile was soft and warm, helping me feel at ease.

"This is the main office of the hospital, next to the front door," she pointed to the room before us with glass sliding windows.

"Mrs Griffiths works there but she is away today and my office is here." She pointed again, this time to a huge door next to the main office on the right. The door had a large brass handle and the words 'Mrs Brunton, Matron' written on a wooden plaque in the centre.

I was to meet Mrs Griffiths in time. She did all the administration and had a huge influence on the running of the whole hospital, from the kitchen staff and the gardener to the matron herself. The hospital couldn't have run without Mrs Griffiths. She also took all the x-rays and ran that department as well.

Mrs Griffiths kept an eagle eye on the financial side of the hospital. I later found out that even pinching a meal off the trolley was almost a sacking offence, although we did risk it at times.

Mrs Brunton took me around to the dining room. She explained about the meals and when and where to order them. You had to write down your order on the pad in the dining room if you wanted a meal, then the cost of the meal would be taken out of your pay. The main meal of the day was at midday and was served to the staff in the dining room. We also had morning and afternoon tea in the dining room. Tea was at 5:30pm and had to be ordered when you came to work in the early afternoon. You could bring your own meal though and have it in the dining room or in the maternity kitchen if you preferred. During the day, you were expected to have all meals and breaks in the dining room. In the evening and at night you could eat in the kitchen located in maternity. There were chairs and tables outside for when the weather was warm and we could have our breaks there.

Mrs Brunton continued giving me the tour. The maternity annexe was at the far end of the hospital. I pondered why she had chosen me to work there. I had not asked to go there but when she rang and asked if I wanted to work in the maternity annexe, I jumped at the chance of working with mothers and babies.

'What a neat job,' I had thought.

As we came to the maternity entrance, there was a door across the other side of the passage, which opened to an outside covered walkway that led to the nurses' home.

On the left was the start of the maternity annexe. As we walked down the corridor, the labour room and connecting bathroom were on the right. The delivery theatre was next to the labour room and, across the corridor from the labour room, was the clean utility where the autoclave machine was kept. The autoclave machine was used to sterilise all the instruments and bowls that were used.

The next room on the right was the dirty utility or pan room and opposite that were the large nursery and the milk room. Along from the milk room, to the left were the staff kitchen, the clean linen room and the dirty linen room.

Next to the nursery, on the other side, was the sisters' office. Mrs Brunton walked into the office and I followed just a few steps behind.

There in the office with her back to us sat a rather large, middle-aged lady with short, grey hair. With a short knock on the door from Mrs Brunton, she turned around.

"Hello hello," she said as she stood up to greet me, making me instantly feel at ease. With her grey hair and short, dumpy appearance, she gave the impression she had been in charge of maternity for a long time.

"Sister Foster, this is Nurse Watts who will be starting here in maternity next week. She has just been measured up for her uniform and I'm giving her a bit of a tour. I think you have her on the roster to start next Monday on the morning shift."

"Welcome to maternity. I'm sure you will enjoy working here. You will be working with one of our more experienced nurses for the first few days so she can show you the ropes. It shouldn't take you too long to settle in," said Sister Foster.

I warmed to Sister Foster the minute I saw her. She had warm, blue eyes and a smile that would, without much provocation, burst into an infectious, raucous laugh. She had devoted her life to a career in midwifery, having had no husband and no family except an elderly mother. She commuted from Woodville, fifteen kilometres away, where she lived with her mother and a cat. I was to learn over the course of time that Mrs Brunton and Sister Foster were not exactly the best of friends, with Sister Foster regularly chucking off at the fact that Mr Brunton was the gardener.

Sister Foster warmly welcomed me onto the staff, explaining shift times and showing me the duty roster for the following fortnight. She gave me a pen and paper so I could write down the shifts that I would be doing for the first two weeks of work.

"This is where the roster is kept and, when you start, we will take you through things. Most of the nurse aides love working here and I'm sure you will like it here as well. Come to the side entrance on Monday morning in time to start at 7am. The door is normally unlocked at that time and if you come to the office here, Nurse Smith will be on shift and she will take you to the changing room."

Both Mrs Brunton and Sister Foster showed me around the rest of the maternity annexe. There were two single rooms for the antenatal women on the left side starting next to the main entrance, then two double rooms before the end of the corridor and the outside door at the other end. On the other side opposite the outside door, there was the patients lounge/dining room. Three double rooms and the patients' toilet and shower were next to the dirty utility room and opposite the sisters' office.

The lino floors were meticulously cleaned and polished thanks to Smithy, the cleaner who worked in maternity. Smithy washed, polished and cleaned the maternity annexe with enthusiasm and gusto. A tall woman in her 50s, Smithy wore a green uniform down past her knees and her hair was short, straight and dark. She wore no makeup and was slightly bent over at the waist leaning to her right side. I knew her as she lived down the road from us in Princess Street.

She greeted me with "Hello, Julie," as we passed in the corridor.

'Nice to see a familiar face,' I thought as we passed her.

The walls were pale green, clean and freshly painted. Not a speck of dust or dirt was to be seen, and the smell of detergent and Savlon was a smell I would come to associate with the hospital and especially maternity.

I was shown the outside door at the end of the corridor and, as I walked down the ramp, I was filled with excitement and expectation for my new job. Not knowing where it would lead or even caring. I was excited just to start.

Born for Life

An Education

THE SHRIEKING RING OF THE alarm clock woke me from a deep sleep. It had taken ages to get to sleep. When I finally did, I was in dreamland. I woke up with a start, and then remembered what today was all about. I lay there for a minute and looked at the clock – 6:00am. All was in darkness as I reluctantly got out of my nice, warm bed. I ran over to the light, switched it on and ran back to where my clothes were laid out. It was freezing and I couldn't get dressed fast enough to try and get warm. I tiptoed out to the kitchen to have some breakfast, shutting the hallway door so as not to disturb anyone.

'Well, this is it,' I thought.

I started to feel so nervous, even to the point of feeling a bit shaky and nauseous. I sat down to eat a bowl of cereal and drink a cup of coffee, savouring every last minute before I had to go. I had packed the flax bag, which I had bought especially for my new job. I had put all my work gear in it the night before. There was a pen, little note book, small scissors, white shoes, stockings and a red cardigan.

I got my lunch from the fridge and thought to myself, 'It's time.'

I sneaked out the front door and carefully closed it so no one would hear me. I braced myself as I walked outside into the icy cold weather. I looked up to see a carpet of white on the lawn lit up by the outside light. Brrr!!! It was freezing. As I got in the car, I noticed the frost on the windscreen. No way could I see through that white frost, so back into the house I went to get a jug of warm water.

That's all I needed, to be late on my first day. I quickly poured the warm water down the windows and ran and put the jug back inside. I was set to go. The car started straight away.

'What a relief.'

I was pleased I didn't have to walk the one-and-a-half kilometres to the hospital in the frost. Barry had lent me his car, a 1955 Mark 1 Consul, so that I could drive to work, which was so sweet of him. He used his motorbike, a 1952 650 BSA, to ride to work. It suited us both, as there was no way I would be able to walk to work in this weather. I would have been numb by the time I got there.

Arriving at the annexe with ten minutes to spare, I slowly got out of the car. I felt anxious as I walked up the ramp to the front door. I went in and walked around to the sisters' office and was met by Betty.

Wearing slippers and her blue cape, I was met with, "Those babies were so unsettled last night that I had to put two of them in the dog box."

Looking through the large nursery window, I saw another room at the end that was the width of the nursery and not very deep, with equipment to one side. One of the babies was still in there. The poor thing had been banished there for crying and disrupting the quiet and peace of the night.

I learnt that most nights, babies would end up in the dog box and even take turns being in there, crying for as long as it took until they eventually fell asleep. The babies would go out to their mothers at feed time and, if they did not settle on their return to the nursery, they would end up in the back room.

Betty showed me the changing room and my locker with my name on it. In the locker were my uniforms and cape with a container full of buttons and clips.

I came out feeling a bit sheepish and was greeted by Frith. Normally there was only one nurse on but, as it was my first day, I had Frith to show me the ropes. Frith had authority and gave an air of superior knowledge. I felt like the new kid on the block and that she was in charge of me. She'd been given the job of teaching me and I could tell she was out to show me a thing or two.

"Come this way," she said in a very commanding tone as she marched off. "We make up the milk first thing so it is ready for the day".

Walking ahead of me she took me into the milk room, which was next to the large nursery where all the babies were kept between feeds. She showed me how to make up the Karilac first, which was essentially sugar and water and given to babies on their first day. I was then shown the formula and how to make that up. Everything went into the fridge, making sure there was enough made up to last the day. There was a chart on the wall by the window with how much a baby would have for its age.

Karilac and water was given for the first day. Half Karilac and half formula milk for the second day. Then full-strength formula milk from the third day. If the baby was breastfed, it had the breast before the Karilac, three minutes on each side per feed on the first day. Then on the second day, five minutes each side and on the third day, ten minutes each side. By then, hopefully the milk would have come in and there would be no need for a complement by the third day.

Regardless of whether the baby was breastfed or bottle fed, the regime was the same. Test weighing the breastfed babies to see how much milk they were getting from their mothers started on day three. Whether the baby needed a complement depended on how much milk the baby got.

"Don't forget to wash your hands before you start," Frith ordered.

There were also small, round trays with lids on and two little, triangular containers inside that were kept in the glass door cabinet. These trays, she told me, were for washing women's nipples before the babies went on the breast. One container was filled with cotton wool and the other was filled with normal saline. The mother would dip some cotton wool in the normal saline and clean the nipples before putting the baby on the breast. The trays were taken out at every feed and brought back to be sterilised afterwards.

Frith's purpose was to show me as much as she could during this shift and, no sooner than the milk had been made up, she marched across the corridor to the dirty utility room. I followed behind, trying to keep up with her and take in as much as I could.

On the right hand side as you walked in was a gleaming, stainless steel bench with a cupboard underneath where the cleaning products and large rolls of cotton wool covered in gauze were kept. Next door to the bench was a large steriliser and another one was on the back wall. The bedpans were kept on wooden racks on the left hand side that went from the back wall to about halfway down the room. There was also a cream, wooden cabinet with glass doors that had loads of glass vases in it.

"We have to clean the stainless steel benches in both the dirty and clean utility rooms every day," Frith instructed.

She then took me next door to the clean utility, which had another shining stainless steel bench and another steriliser. Underneath the bench was a cupboard with a large container inside that was also made of stainless steel. A plastic container of used soap sat beside it.

"This is the soap for the enemas," she said, bringing out the large container filled with a jelly-like substance.

"You make up the enema mixture with the used soap and boiling water, letting the soap dissolve and then mixing it up. The soap then sets like this jelly and we use it for the enemas." I remained silent while she continued to explain, as I had no idea what she was talking about.

Frith then took me through the labour room and into the bathroom next to it. The room had a bath and a hand basin with a toilet by the bath. The bath was covered with a board and made up into a bed with a pillow on top.

From the cupboard under the hand basin she produced a round, narrow, stainless steel container with a long, brown, hollow tube coming out from the bottom. She explained that a good tablespoon of the soap went into the container and you then filled the container up with warm water, dissolving the jellied soap. The end of the tube was put into the woman's anus, or back passage, and you held the container up so all the liquid went into the rectum.

"Don't pull out the tube until all the fluid is in the body. Then you keep the woman lying on her side until she needs to go to the toilet and stand clear," Frith said. "That normally gets them going and they have a good crap."

I felt very naïve, as I had never heard of half of what she was telling me. I had never even heard the word bowel or enema in all my sixteen years. I was learning some very adult stuff, very fast.

Frith then showed me a stainless steel tray with some liquid soap and a razor in a bowl and some cotton wool in another small bowl. There were also packets of gloves in the cupboard and a trumpet-shaped vase-like thing that was hollow and narrow at one end, wide at the other and made of aluminium. Frith told me this was a pinard for listening to the baby's heartbeat through the mother's abdomen.

When a woman came into the maternity annexe in labour, I was to bring her into this bathroom first and call the sister. The woman was then prepared for labour. She had to have all her pubic hair shaved, an enema, blood pressure taken and an examination by the sister. After a clean out in the toilet, the board with the mattress and bed on it was removed and the woman had a warm bath before going into the labour room.

Depending on the examination and assessment by the sister, the woman, if in advanced labour, would proceed into the delivery theatre where the nurse on duty or I would call the doctor when the sister told us to. Otherwise, the woman was to stay in the labour room until she was ready to have her baby and then she would go into the theatre. In early labour the woman was allowed to walk around.

The father was allowed into the labour room but not into the theatre and was to wait outside until the baby was born. Then when the doctor had finished what needed to be done, like suturing and the examination of the baby, the mother and baby were wheeled back into the labour room, where the new mum and dad could have a cup of tea and some toast before the mother was wheeled down to a postnatal room.

For the delivery in theatre, the only people allowed in were the doctor, the sister and the nurse aide. All had to wear white gowns down to the ground, theatre hats that covered all our hair and masks.

My mind was exploding with all this information as we came out of the labour room and into the corridor. I could see Sister Foster had made a cup of tea in the kitchen, which she was about to take into the office.

"Well, hello. I hope Frith is showing you around and explaining everything to you." she said, smiling at me.

Frith then led me into the office and showed me a folder with all the duties for the various shifts and the times to do each task. It was something to refer to if I forgot the routine, I thought with relief.

There was no rooming-in, so all the babies were kept in the nursery, not in the room with their mother. The babies were on strict four hourly feeding so the mother had to have a fantastic milk supply to fully breastfeed. As a nurse aide, just out of school and with no training, I was expected to assist the women with breastfeeding and help put the baby on the breast. The sister would also assist if she was not otherwise engaged.

The visitors, including the fathers and family, had to look at their baby through the nursery window. At visiting time, the bell rang for everyone to come and have a look at the baby they wanted to see. The nurse aide would go into the nursery and lift up each baby at the window to show the friends and relatives.

I started to feel overwhelmed by what was expected of me and wondered if I was up to the job. However, I hardly had time to even think about it, Frith continued with the task at hand and showed me more of what I was expected to do.

It was nearly time to prepare for bath time in the nursery. After the bath, it was the babies' feed time. I followed Frith into the nursery and she proceeded to show me what needed to be done. The baths were filled up with warm water and all the clothes, nappies and towels for bath time were put out in bundles.

The babies were all in their cribs in the nursery and the mothers were called when it was their baby's turn for a bath. The first day we showed the mother how it was done and then she was expected to bath the baby on her own after that. Mothers stayed in for about five to seven days, so were very familiar with caring for their baby by the time they went home.

It was my first day too and, since I had never held a baby before, Frith showed me and a new mum how it was done. Once the baby was bathed, the mother wheeled her baby to her room for feed time, taking a bottle from the milk room if needed.

Once all the babies were out, we would clean the cribs and change the linen. We filled the bottom of the cribs with bundles of nappies and extra clothes, consisting of a singlet, gown and a cuddly rug. Sister Foster poked her head in to see how it was going and then ambled down the corridor to the rooms to see if any of the mothers needed a hand with breastfeeding. Sister Foster was never one for being hands on, but gave advice while she was observing. Frith and I also popped in to see the mothers to see how the feeding was going. I just followed Frith's lead. We then cleaned the nursery, which included cleaning the baby baths, damp dusting all the benches and surfaces, mopping the floors and cleaning the stainless steel benches and hand basin.

It was an hour before all the babies were fed and back in the nursery.

"It's morning tea time," Frith announced when all the babies were back.

I could tell Frith was keen for a break and so was I, for that matter. I needed time out from all the information I was getting. I was sure I would never remember it all. We made our way down the corridor to the dining room. Both of us poured a cup of tea and, taking a scone, we looked around for somewhere to sit. The big table at the end of the room had Mrs Griffiths, Mrs Sinclair and the sisters from the general ward around it.

The nurse aides sat around the smaller tables that were scattered around the room, while the cleaning and kitchen staff (greenies) sat at the other end by the door. We made our way over to where some other nurses were sitting.

"Hi, I'm Linda," the little nurse with dark hair said as I sat down. "I started here three months ago, working in general," she continued.

I learnt that Linda came from a farming family, was living in the nurses' home and went home on her days off.

"Hi, I'm Julie and it's my first day today," I said.

"This is Ann, who works mainly in theatre and sometimes in general," said Linda, as she tried to help me feel at ease.

I knew Ann, a nurse aide who had worked at the hospital for years and was well regarded. I recognized a few of the staff from around town over at the greenies' table. They were mostly older women who did the cleaning and cooking at the hospital.

I found out later that a few girls from school had also started working in maternity or would start soon. There was Debbie, who was from my year at school, but in the class above mine. There was Jane and Christine, who were both a year older than me. Marcia, my best friend from college, also joined the maternity staff soon after me and lived in the nurses' home because she was from a farm near Eketahuna.

The dining room was a hub of activity, especially in the mornings when morning tea was supplied in the form of scones, sandwiches or toasted sandwiches – all made by the kitchen staff. A large pot of tea was made and put on the bench for everyone. If you wanted coffee, then you made your own.

"Can you show me how to order my dinner before we go back?" I asked Linda while we were chatting.

"Sure. I normally have a hot dinner when I'm on a morning shift. I live in the nurses' home, so it's the only hot meal I'll get. I don't cook that much over there. A large, heated, stainless steel trolley gets brought around to the dining room at about 11:30am, so from then on you can come around to get your dinner. The trolley is heated so it's warm no matter what time you get here."

"Thanks for that. I'm just trying to find out as much as I can about how it all works."

"Look, I will try and get here around twelve o'clock if Sister says I can go and I'll meet you then. Not much fun eating on your own."

"That would be great. I'll see if I can get here then. It all depends on Frith and Sister Foster though."

We finished our break and Frith and I walked back to maternity.

"You know, we have got the best deal in maternity. A lot of the girls in general are so envious of us. They think we have it so cushy in maternity and we do," Frith said.

It didn't take long to work out what she was meaning. The

maternity staff felt a bit superior to the general staff in a way and the general staff felt we had it sweet in maternity. After all, we were dealing with a lovely stage of life – the birth of a baby – and caring for lovely babies and their mothers. Mostly it was happy families.

The general staff, on the other hand, were dealing with sick people who were often old and sometimes incontinent. They also had dementia patients who would often throw things around and abuse them. They were, on the whole, a lot busier than us. We had time to talk to the mothers and it was a lovely place to work.

I felt privileged to be working in the nicest part of the hospital, although there were challenges – as young girls, we had responsibilities well beyond our years, although initially I didn't realise how much. We were never trained, as such, but learnt on the job and were given instructions from the sisters. We never questioned what we were doing or why we were doing it. We just followed their orders and were under their authority.

Despite Firth's forthright manner and bossy way of telling me things, she did appear to know what she was talking about and seemed very experienced. At least she was giving me as much information as she could, because soon I would be on my own and only have the sister to ask.

Born for Life

An Almighty Push

I HAD BEEN WORKING FOR a week when I arrived for my shift in the early afternoon and the two sisters were in the office. There was Sister Drury for the morning duty and Sister Foster for the afternoon. Debbie, the morning nurse, filled me in on what was happening with the mothers and babies who were in. The nurse aides gave the report to each other at the change of shift and the sisters did the same. We always handed over to each other in the kitchen, while the sisters handed over to one another in the office.

As I passed the labour room on my way to get changed, I noticed there was some activity in the room and then realised there was someone in labour. I started to get nervous and I could feel myself becoming anxious, thinking that I would be on my own with the sister for the afternoon shift. I had never had a shift when there was a woman in labour before.

I went and rang the bell for the visitors to come and see the babies in the nursery. They all came and pointed to the baby they wanted to see. Very carefully, I lifted up the end of the crib, making sure that the face of the baby was seen. After they slowly dispersed, Debbie and I made afternoon tea for the sisters and took it to them on a tray. After knocking on the open door and after receiving a "come in", I put the tray on the desk.

"Thank you, Nurse," said Sister Drury.

"Can we go to afternoon tea now?" I asked.

"Yes, that will be fine."

"Come on, Deb. Let's go," I called as I walked past the kitchen and headed for the dining room.

We poured ourselves a cup of tea and went outside. Deb lit up a cigarette and offered me one. I took it and lit up.

"You'll be right with Mrs Little. She's all prepped and has got going. Probably round six o'clock she'll have it," Deb said as she started to sit down.

"Is that the one in labour? What do I do? I've never had anyone in labour before." I was beginning to panic. 'WHAT DO I DO?' I thought, as I felt my heart pounding.

"Just go in there and rub her back and do anything else she wants. Sister Foster will tell you what to do." Debbie seemed so calm, like nothing would faze her.

My palms started to sweat and I felt a cold shiver come over me. Even though I wanted to run, I knew I had to face this at some point and there was no getting out of it. There was a woman in labour on my shift and I had to deal with it.

On returning, I gingerly and nervously entered the labour room after Debbie had gone. I was like a little child again, going to school for the first time, as if I was entering into a great unknown.

Loud breathing noises were coming from Mrs Little, with periods of normal breathing. She lay on the bed facing the wall. I went and stood by the bed, observing and not knowing if she even knew I was standing there. Again it would come, "huh huh whew, huh huh whew, huh huh whew," she breathed as she closed her eyes, grasping the bed sheets and moving her legs in the bed. After about a minute, it ended and she reached for a glass of water. I handed it to her. "Thank you" was her only response and then she rested.

In the kitchen, Sister Foster was sitting at the table reading the paper and having a smoke.

"Come and get me when she wants to push or if you see any anal pouting."

"Is she alright?" I asked.

"Yes, she's fine. I'll be in soon to take her blood pressure. You go back in there and call me if you need me. She might like you to rub her back."

I went back in the room and the tension and pain on Mrs Little's face was something I had never seen before. 'This must be serious pain,' I thought. "Would you like me to rub your back?" I asked.

Turning so her back faced me, she pulled up the hospital nightie she had on. Mr Little was standing at the end of the room looking like a helpless, lost soul. I looked over at the packed suitcase beside him, as he stood over at the end of the room looking as if he didn't know where to put himself. I got the spare chair and put it beside the head of the bed.

"Would you like to sit here?" I asked trying to help him feel at ease.

"Thanks. I just need to go out for a smoke. Will be back in a minute," he answered.

I sat down between the wall and the bed and started rubbing Mrs Little's back. It was difficult to rub on bare skin, so I put the nightie between my hand and her skin. She was so hot and sticky with perspiration.

"Huh huh whew, huh huh whew," began again and I started to rub again.

"Lower down, lower down," she cried out.

My hand moved down to the lower back just above the buttocks. There was another rest and then again, "huh huh whew." The same pattern repeated over and over for what must have been at least an hour.

Sister Foster ambled in after about an hour. I moved out of the way while she took her blood pressure. She then got the woman to turn on her back, while she felt her large, swollen tummy. Then, taking the pinard, listened to the baby's heartbeat, with her ear at the narrow end, while the wide end was pressed firmly against Mrs Little's lower tummy.

Then, I saw her whole abdomen rise up and become like a hard tight ball.

"Oh no," was the cry, "not again, huh huh whew," as Mrs Little turned back on her side.

"Just let me know when the contraction has finished, as I want to examine you and see how far along you are," explained the sister.

Turning to me, Sister asked, "Nurse, can you go and start changing the babies for the five o'clock feed and take them out while I do this? Then come back here when they are all out."

I hesitated, curious as to what the examination involved. Sister put a glove on her right hand and put some white cream on her fingers. I was astounded to see her put her finger up Mrs Little's back passage. She appeared to be moving her finger around inside, before removing them.

'How strange,' I thought.

"You are about seven centimetres and the cervix is thinning out nicely." She then replaced the covers as I went out to start getting the babies ready for feed time.

As I started changing the first baby, a tinge of excitement came over me, 'I am going to see a baby born,' I thought to myself. I hurriedly took the babies out one by one, so I could get back into the labour room as quick as I could.

I had become quite good at changing nappies. I would undo the pin and see what was inside. If it was wet, I would undo a new nappy bundle and lay it under the baby. There was a triangular nappy next to the baby and another nappy, which had one corner folded down, underneath the triangular one. I took the first side of the triangular nappy over the body, then the other side and then brought up the bit in the middle and secured it with a safety pin. The second nappy was then wrapped around the legs.

I brought the singlet and gown down and then folded it back up so the baby would not wet it. If the nappy had black tar stuff called meconium, which was the newborns' bowel motions for the first two or three days, then in the large stainless steel drums on the centre bench were material squares that were used to wash the dirty bottom. In another large drum, material squares had Vaseline smeared on them, which were folded over and then used to put on the little bottom so the meconium would not stick to the skin. We would fill the containers and fold the nappy bundles in our quiet times and on night duty.

One by one, I changed the babies and took them out to their mothers. I carried them out rather than taking them in their cribs, as I thought it would be quicker. The last baby was out when I remembered the breast trays and the bottles. All four babies were breastfed so four trays were needed. One needed the Karilac and one needed half formula and half Karilac. The other two were fully breastfeeding.

I had just got all that done when I remembered, 'Oh no, I forgot to test weigh the two that were fully breastfed.'

I was tempted to leave it, but wouldn't dare to, so I rushed back to the room and got one of the babies. The mother had just started pulling her nightie up.

"Sorry, I forgot the test weigh," I said as I grabbed the baby, taking it back to the nursery.

I then put the baby, fully clothed, on the scales, scribbled the weight down on a hand towel beneath its name and then took the baby back to its mother. Fully breastfed babies were test weighed every second day from day three. We weighed before the feed and again after the feed. The weight difference was the amount of milk the baby had received. How much the baby received determined if they needed a top up of formula.

"Ten minutes each side now. Can you manage on your own?" I asked.

"I'm ok," was the reply. Relieved, I then went and got the other baby and repeated the exercise. All the babies were now out, so I quickly went back to the labour room.

Sister Foster was still there. "Let me know if she starts pushing or if you see any anal pressure."

"What?" I asked.

She repeated herself and said "I'll get the babies back in. Dr Symes should be in soon so come and get me when he comes." Daring not to ask what she meant, I started rubbing Mrs Little's back again.

"Can it please stop? I want to die," she cried.

All I could say was, "It will be ok" and then I thought, 'I hope it will be ok and that she doesn't die.'

I then heard a deep, gruff cough and the sound of loud footsteps. Into the room came Dr Symes. I knew him as he was my doctor. There were only two general practitioners in town, so they were both well known and recognized. I would even say he had a god-like presence.

"Is Sister here?" he asked.

"I'll go and get her," I said and rushed away to find Sister Foster, hoping she was not too far away.

"Dr Symes has arrived," I said when I found her in one of the rooms.

"Can you take Baby Grant and Baby Smith back to the nursery," she instructed as she set off down the corridor to the labour room.

After getting the babies back and emptying the nappy bucket into the linen bag, I waited in the kitchen, feeling it was not my place to enter the labour room while the door was closed. After about ten minutes, I heard heavy footsteps walk down the corridor and go out the main door.

Sister Foster came into the kitchen.

"She's not far away now, so call me if you need me. His Lordship is going home now. If we need him, the phone number is on the sheet by the phone outside theatre. I'll be in the office. Just ring the bell."

Sister Foster always referred to the doctors as 'His Lordship' behind their backs. I was always amused when she said it.

I went back into the labour room. The pain seemed to be more intense now and my back rubbing did not seem to cut it anymore.

Mrs Little was rolling around the bed due to the contractions and seemed out of control. All I could do was hold her hand now. Her husband came around to her other side and held her other hand. Seemingly helpless, but giving encouraging words all the same.

"Oh oh, mmm huh huh huh mmmm," she groaned. "Oh no I've wet myself," said Mrs Little as she rolled her head from side to side on the pillow.

Looking down, I could see a large pool of straw coloured fluid. The contractions were so strong, I felt afraid of what was happening.

Rushing out, I called, "Sister, Sister. Please come quick." Sister Foster appeared and came into the room hurriedly.

"Open that double door," she summoned, indicating the door that led into theatre. While helping move the bed out assisted by Mr Little, I opened the double doors. Sister Foster and I wheeled the bed into theatre and transferred Mrs Little onto the narrow theatre bed. I wheeled the labour bed back into the labour room, leaving poor Mr Little standing in the labour room as I shut the door again.

"Right, put this gown and cap on, Nurse. Here is a mask. Well, it shouldn't be long now as her waters have now gone."

"Undo that bundle on the trolley, Nurse. Don't touch anything inside as it's sterile."

'Well, ok,' I thought, as I started ripping the tape off the bundle. I had been told what to do here, but had never done it before. As I gently and carefully undid the bundle, daring not to touch anything inside, I looked down at my shaking hands.

"Take the tongs in that container and spread the linen to the back of the trolley and the instruments and bowls to the front." I heard as Sister kept giving me instructions while she stood at the end of the bed.

I carefully did what I was told. Whew, I felt so relieved that I had not dropped anything on the floor or touched anything with my hands. I glanced around. Sister was wiping the fluid away from Mrs Little's private area and had a pad in place. Mrs Little had a hospital gown on and a cuddly had been put over her lower body.

"Put some warm Savlon in that big bowl and some obstetric cream in the smaller one," Sister said, pointing to the trolley I had just set up.

"We'll see what's happening here." Sister then dipped a large gauze pad into the Savlon and wiped Mrs Little's whole bottom area, from the remaining pubic hair to the anus.

"Now when she gets another contraction, I want you to hold her leg up," she said, indicating for me to come around to the side of Mrs Little.

She walked around to the foot of the bed, leaving me at the side with Mrs Little's back facing me. There seemed to be a longer period now between each contraction and we seemed to be almost waiting for them to happen. At least I felt I could catch my breath and calm myself while we were waiting for the next contraction to come.

I could see Sister Foster with a needle and glass syringe. She drew up some fluid from the glass vial, put the syringe into a small kidney dish and put it on the little table at the head of the bed.

"Now, Nurse, when I tell you, I want you to take the syringe and needle and put it into her leg here. Wait until I tell you. Wipe the leg first with this swab, put the needle in her leg and then slowly push the plunger down until all the fluid has gone."

"Mmmmuh, mmmmuh, mmmmmuh." I looked over to see Mrs

Little, red faced, tense and straining like she was on the toilet doing a poo.

"Lift the leg so I can see," Sister said, pointing to the upper leg as she stood on the opposite side. I duly lifted the leg as the next contraction came.

A quick breath and again came the "mmmmmuh, mmmmuh, mmmmuh."

"Push, push, push," called Sister. I glanced down and could see nothing. I was wondering what it was that I was going to see.

"That one is over. Put the leg down," said Sister. There was another break of about four minutes and time for us all to relax a bit.

A look at Mrs Little's face told it all. I went and got a flannel, wet it with cold water and wiped her face. Beads of perspiration dotted her forehead and her face was red down to the neck. She lay on her left side and I lifted her upper leg with every contraction as soon as it started. I could see her face and, every time I saw the pain in her face, that was my cue. Sister brought around a large cylinder with a tube attached and a mask at the end that went over Mrs Little's face. She gave it to Mrs Little to breathe into every time a contraction came.

"Have some gas but not too much. Just two puffs, then hold your breath and push as if you need your bowels to move."

"Imagine you are constipated and having the biggest bowel motion ever," Sister said.

Whenever the contraction came, the mask would be given, the leg would go up and Sister would just keep yelling, "Push, push, push," and then "that's the way – hold your breath and PUSH."

I worked up the courage to look down while I held the leg high

32

and slightly bent. I could see the anus pouting out and, 'Oh, gross,' I thought. 'There is some poo coming out.'

Sister had some toilet paper at the ready and wiped the poo away after every contraction. The pushing continued for about thirty minutes. I was getting more confident at looking at her anus and vagina.

"I can't do it, I can't do it. I want to die. CUT IT OUT," she screamed.

Sister then got angry and started telling Mrs Little, "Stop it and just push. Look, I can see the baby's head."

With that, I looked down and there was some hair just coming out of the bulging perineum. 'I can't believe this,' I thought. 'Wow, is that the head? It must be,' I thought.

"Mmmmmuh, mmmmmuh, mmmmmuh," came with every contraction and the vagina started opening up more and more.

'It is just like having a big poo,' I thought 'and the more she pushes, the more the anus and poo comes out. But also, the vagina is opening up and stretching and more of the head is coming. Wow!'

I started to feel I had a role to play in this baby coming into the world. I felt important that I had a role, even if it was just lifting a leg and wiping a hot, sweaty face. With each push came progress, little by little, and more and more of the head was visible. Even Mrs Little seemed to be more into it and stopped wanting to die, which I thought must be good.

Sister Foster stopped being angry and seemed happy that the baby was slowly coming out.

"Now, when I tell you, go to the phone outside and ring Dr Symes. Tell him that Mrs Little is ready for delivery and then come back. Also, go down to the main door and make sure it is unlocked," instructed Sister.

"Alright," I said, going over in my head what I had to say and do.

As the pushing continued, I noticed more fluid coming out of the vagina and saw some blood as well. The part of the head that I could see was about an egg cup in size when I got the word to go and call the doctor. I rushed out, nervously picked up the phone and dialled the number.

"Mrs Little is ready for delivery," I said and then, without waiting for a response, hung up and rushed out to check the door.

When I came back, Mrs Little was on her back, sitting up slightly and continuing to push.

"Put these gloves on," Sister said, pointing to a box of gloves on the wall.

It was getting so hot with the mask on that I wanted to take it off so I could breathe. I knew I couldn't do that, so every now and then I would try and let some fresh air in by pulling it out a bit. It seemed like no time at all before I heard the heavy, loud footsteps of the doctor. You could not mistake the cough as well. I could hear him putting on one of the aprons that were hanging on the hooks outside the door and taking his shoes off to put on the white gumboots that were lined up in a row under the aprons.

As he entered the theatre, I could see his large, dark-rimmed glasses starting to steam over.

'Must be cold outside,' I thought.

Going over to the basin to wash his hands, he turned to Sister and asked, "How long has she been pushing, Sister?"

"About an hour and a half now," came the reply. He went over to the trolley, dried his hands with a towel, got a green gown and started putting it on, turning for Sister to tie it up at the back. He then put on the gloves that were on the trolley.

"Can you wipe my glasses please, Sister?" he asked, turning to face Sister Foster.

"Well you have done really well, Emma," he said, looking at Mrs Little. "Let me see a few good pushes now."

"Ok," was the reply. Mrs Little seemed to get some energy and encouragement from the doctor's presence. With that, another contraction came. With her head down and using all her might, Mrs Little gave an almighty push. I could see even more of the head now and the vagina had stretched out so that it was tight against the baby's head. The head seemed to be pushing through.

For the next fifteen minutes the contractions kept coming and Mrs Little continued to push as hard as she could.

"We might have to do a cut to help the baby out, Emma," said Dr Symes.

Next thing, I saw him take a syringe out of a cloth that Sister had placed on the trolley and he attached a needle to it.

"Could I have some local, Sister?" and with that Sister got a small bottle from the drawer and held it upside down, while Dr Symes put the needle into the bottle and drew up all the liquid inside. As the baby's head started coming with the next contraction, Dr Symes inserted his fingers by the baby's head. He injected the needle into the edge of the perineum and emptied the contents of the syringe.

"The baby will come with the next contraction, Emma. Not long now."

I then saw the doctor take a pair of scissors, which were bent at the blades. With his fingers inside the vagina and next to the baby's head, he put one of the scissor blades in and cut a large piece of flesh. In shock, I stared at the gaping wound and then at the woman, expecting her to scream out with pain.

Apart from the pain she was already in, she didn't seem to be aware. Next thing, as I looked at the baby, the whole head gradually emerged, looking all wet and blue. Its eyes were closed and fluid was coming out of the baby's mouth. Doctor Symes' large, gloved hands were on the baby's head as Sister wiped its head and face with a dry gauze cloth.

As the next contraction came, the hands on the baby's head slowly pulled down and the baby's body slid out of its mother's. I had just seen my very first birth.

All Gowned Up

IT WAS THE WEEKEND AND all of my family had gone out to the bach. Because I was rostered to work on Saturday afternoon and Sunday morning, I was unable to go. It was the first time that I had missed going out to the beach with them. Dad had built the bach in 1963, assisted by his brother Doug and Grandad, when I was ten years old. It was out at Mataikona, which was on the Wairarapa Coast an hour's drive from Masterton. Once built, every time there was a free weekend, public holiday or opportunity for Dad to escape his florist business, we headed for the bach. It was a haven that I relished from the age of ten – a retreat and a paradise – although this weekend work had to come first.

I couldn't help thinking about what fun they might be having as I drove to work. I was on duty with Sister Drury, whom I had never worked with before. She was very friendly, although she was sarcastic at times, which left you wondering, 'Did she mean that or was she joking?'

She spent a lot of time in the office stuffing dolls, which she sewed at home and brought to work for when it was quiet. They were rag dolls with long limbs and made of different coloured materials.

It seemed she had plenty of orders for the dolls and was kept very busy. She was a Maori midwife who came up from Masterton to work. She would stay at the nurses' home when she was working a few shifts on the trot. When she stayed, she was also on call for the night shift. There was a nurse on the ward for the night shift and the sisters took turns at being on call, sleeping in the nurses' home.

After we had afternoon tea and the morning staff had gone home, I went to see Sister Drury in the office.

"Have you done a perineal toilet before?" she asked.

"Well no, not yet," I replied.

She explained that for the first 24 hours after a birth, women were in bed, so we had to toilet them and wash their perineum down to keep the area clean. This was done every four hours. After the 24 hours, they were allowed to get up, walk around as normal, and go to the toilet by themselves. We had to get them up and assist them for their first shower the next morning, like an initiation back to normal bathroom activities.

"Come and get me at 4pm when Mrs Butler is ready for her swab and I'll show you how to do one," she said.

I started preparing the trolley for the swab just before the time it was due. I had seen a trolley prepared before so had an idea of what needed to go on it. I got the stainless steel trolley out and started putting things on it. I got two pans and pan covers down and put them on the bottom of the trolley. I then grabbed clean linen, a clean draw sheet, a binder, a material pad, two normal pads and a perineal toilet pack. I remembered that when I had seen other nurses coming back from doing swabs, they were wearing gowns and masks, so I quickly went and got a gown and put it on along with a mask.

"I'm ready, Sister," I called, as I started to wheel the trolley down the corridor to the room. Sister Drury followed closely behind.

As we walked into the room, Sister Drury announced, "It's that time again, Mrs Butler. It's the first time Nurse has done a perineal toilet so I am here to show her how it's done."

Mrs Butler lay down and started undoing the pins that held the binder together. I put some gloves on before I took all the bloody linen away, put it on the bottom of the trolley and put the first pan under her buttocks.

"Right, now Nurse, when she has passed urine you need to take that pan away, put it under the trolley, get the other pan and put that one under her. Then go and wash your hands and put some sterile gloves on. You should undo the pack first before you start washing your hands."

I gingerly took the nearly full pan of urine and, trying not to spill it, put it under the trolley. I then took the new pan and put it under Mrs Butler's bottom, hoping she could not see how nervous I was. I tried not to think too much about how embarrassed I felt. I was sure Mrs Butler would be feeling embarrassed as well, being all exposed like this and peeing with two people standing over her.

'Not very comfortable, I'm sure. What a messy business,' I thought.

I went over to the basin and washed my hands.

As I finished, Sister Drury continued, "Come on, Nurse. Get over here. Now put these gloves on. Look, you have forgotten the sterile bowl and to get the warm Savlon and put it into a sterile jug. You are all scrubbed now so I'll have to go and get it."

With that, Sister went off in a real huff. I could hear her banging around all the way down in the utility room. I stood all gowned and gloved up with my hands in the air unable to touch anything. All dressed up but nowhere to go, waiting for her to return.

"Here it is," she said as she put the bowl and the jug of Savlon on the trolley. She then instructed me to pour some of the Savlon into the bowl.

'Fortunately I have this mask on to hide my red face,' I thought.

Sister Drury then started pushing down on Mrs Butler's stomach. I looked at Mrs Butler's face as she grimaced at the discomfort she was enduring.

"You have to rub up the fundus like this after they have passed urine," she said continuing to push down really hard with her hand, seemingly oblivious to Mrs Butler's discomfort and crying out. I noticed more blood coming out from the vagina when she stopped rubbing and the instructions continued.

"Now take those forceps, pick up some cotton wool and dip it in the Savlon. Wipe the cotton wool down the perineum from the front to the back and then drop the cotton wool in the pan. Don't go from back to front, it must be from front to back."

Sister Drury stood on the other side peering down at what I was doing.

"Ok," I said as I started doing what I was told. I was ever so careful, as I was worried I would push too hard and hurt Mrs Butler.

"Now when you have done that a few times, take the jug of warm Savlon and pour it down the perineum, then dry the area with the rest of the cotton wool," Sister Drury continued. "Now take the pan away and we'll change this linen."

I could tell she was getting a bit impatient with showing me what to do, so I quickly took the pan away and put the pads in place.

Sister starting pulling out the dirty draw sheet on her side and pushed it towards the middle of the bed. She then took the clean one and tucked it into the side of the bed and, rolling Mrs Butler over to me, she laid out the clean draw sheet. She rolled Mrs Butler back again to get the dirty draw sheet out.

"Take the dirty draw sheet out from your side, Nurse, and straighten up the clean sheet. Now get the pads and put them in place, then put the binder like this under her back and bring it around like this as tight as you can. The tighter the better so she can get her figure back."

With that, Sister Drury got the binder that she had laid under Mrs Butler's back and pulled it with all her might, bringing it over Mrs Butler's stomach and pinning it with the safety pins. I looked at Mrs Butler and she seemed to be ok with it all. Once she was pinned, she looked all bound up like an Egyptian mummy, but didn't seem uncomfortable or in pain at all. She then slowly sat up in bed.

I wheeled the trolley back to the dirty utility room, where I unpacked all the dirty linen and rubbish from the procedure. I looked at the clock.

'Golly, 4:40pm already, nearly time to start changing the babies for the next feed,' I thought and then went into the nursery to start. There were only three mothers and babies in, so it wasn't too busy and this gave me a chance to get confident with everything I had to do. Sister Drury followed me in.

"Make sure that you wash your hands between every baby, Nurse," she said as I started unwrapping one of the babies.

Everything still felt new, from the environment and the routine, to caring for mothers and babies – and everything in between. Being only sixteen years old, it seemed overwhelming at times.

Every day was different, as I was fast finding out. Each day there were new challenges to face. At the change of each shift there was the chance to talk to the nurse coming on about things I was unsure of. When I was working a morning shift, I was on my own with the sister and Smithy once the other nurse left. On the afternoon shift, another greenie would come on around 5pm, give out the tea, collect all the dishes, wash them and then go home.

Then there was learning the hierarchy, the order of people, what was expected of you and what everyone else did. You weren't exactly told, but somehow you picked it up along the way. Although you were certainly told if you got it wrong. That was something I had to get used to – being told what to do and being treated like a servant. Everyone had a place and a position. You only addressed people by their first name if they were the same position as you or lower, otherwise you addressed them by their title.

I changed the babies and, one by one, started taking them out to their mothers. Sister Drury went back in the office.

She left me to get the babies out on my own and went and checked on how the mothers were going with feeding once the babies were out.

Most of the sisters would help when we needed it, otherwise they left us to it and would go around the mothers at some stage to check on how the feeding was going and give advice.

Both feed times for the 5pm and the 9pm feeds went well. One of the mothers who had been in for three days had very engorged breasts, which seemed to be quite common. The feed times were strictly four hourly and if the baby had not taken enough milk, the breasts soon became sore and engorged. Sister Drury had gone down to see a woman when she rang the bell at the 9pm feed and asked me to get a breast binder organised. Since I hadn't done that before, she came down to the utility room to show me how to prepare a breast binder.

She showed me the large squares of cotton wool with gauze on the outside. Two of the squares had to have a hole cut in the middle for the nipple to fit through. We folded the squares twice, then cut off a corner to create a square in the middle once unfolded, which is where the nipple went. These squares were put onto the hot steriliser and had oil poured around most of the square, but not where it was cut. They were then left on the sterilizer until the oil become warm and the cotton wool was all puffed up.

Sister asked me to ring the bell when I was down in the room and ready to put the binder on, so she could show me how it went. Mrs Evans lay down and took her nightie off. Her breasts were like large, shining beacons. They were enormous and the skin looked so tight, as if they would pop if they were pricked with a pin. They looked so red and sore.

Sister Drury arrived, "Ok, put the oiled gauze square on the breast, making sure the nipple can go through the hole you've cut. Make sure they aren't too hot. The last thing Mrs Evans needs is burnt breasts, so nice and warm but not too hot. Then put the plain gauze square without the oil over the oiled one. Take a folded nappy and put that over the cotton wool pads, then the breast binder can be put on. The binder is wrapped around the back and then comes around to the front, pulled together and pinned like the abdominal binder. Then take the two straps that came from the back and bring them over the shoulders and pin them at the front to hold the binder up."

I followed the instructions closely and was relieved when the job was done and the breasts were bound up and put away.

"Alright, that looks nice and firm. Thank you for showing me. I'll be able to do it next time," I said as Sister left the room.

I had just finished putting in the last pin when we heard the phone ring.

"That's the phone," Sister Drury called out as she went up to the office to answer it.

I was in the nursery putting the last baby down to sleep when Sister Drury came into the nursery.

"Nurse, could you please get the prep room ready as we've got someone coming in – in labour."

I finished putting the baby down, went into the prep room and got out the tray with the razor and stainless steel bowls on. I put some Savlon in one bowl, some liquid soap in the other and then got out the container to mix up the soap and water enema. I left it on the locker along with the other tray.

I had no sooner come out of the prep room when Mrs Morris and her husband arrived. I took her into the labour room to drop her bag off and then went into the prep room, giving her husband a seat to sit on while he was waiting.

"We shouldn't be too long, Mr Morris. If you can wait here for a bit while we prep your wife." I thrust a pile of magazines into his hand.

Mrs Morris followed me into the prep room.

"Sister will be in shortly," I said. "Can you please put this gown on? Just put all your other clothes in the labour room."

I left her to undress and put the nightie on and came out to the office.

"I'll go and prep her, Nurse. You might as well go home when the night nurse comes on, as you are on again in the morning."

"Thank you, Sister," I said looking at the clock. Where had the time gone? It was nearly the end of the shift. Betty arrived soon after. I told her what had gone on that shift and about the new woman who was in the prep room.

Betty was the regular night nurse doing five shifts a week. She had two daughters who did lots of activities after school, so it was nothing for Betty to work a night shift and then have to go to something that was on for her daughters during the day. She seemed to survive on very little sleep, but did things at work in the quiet times like sewing her daughters' costumes for their ballet recitals. She brought two great big bags to work with her that were filled with all her projects.

She was very talkative and hard to get away from most nights when she arrived. She chattered about everything from her daughters and how well they were doing, to what was going on at the hospital and what a pain her husband was. In her eyes, he seemed to cause her endless grief. I liked her company though and would often get talking and find I still had not left the hospital at 11:30pm.

I was going to go straight home tonight though, since I was working again in the morning. After giving handover, I quickly went and got changed.

"Bye, I'll see you in the morning," I said as I headed out the door.

'Brrrr . . . another cold night but hopefully not a frost,' I thought as I walked down the ramp to the car.

Fortunately, I still had Barry's car to use. It was a long-term loan so long as I kept going out with him, I presumed. I don't know how

I would have managed without it. I suppose I would have had to buy my own car, but the thought had never crossed my mind. I was happy with the current arrangement.

Quiet Please

NEXT MORNING I WOKE WITH the alarm, showered, had breakfast and was back at the maternity annexe. As I walked in, there was an eerie quiet, or something different that I couldn't put my finger on. The atmosphere was not usual. No one was in sight, so I went to get changed. As I walked past the labour room I noticed that it was empty, but all the doors were open to the delivery room. I got a glimpse of it being in disarray, needing to be cleaned and put back together. The bed was still stripped and the delivery trolley looked as if it had been used. I came out of the changing room and, as I was coming down the corridor, I saw Betty. She motioned for me to go into the kitchen where she followed and shut the door. I stood, bracing myself for what she was going to say, as her face was one of sheer anxiety.

"Something terrible has happened," she said.

"Mrs Morris had an eclamptic fit last night," she continued. "She delivered the baby very quickly. We got her into the delivery room alright and the birth went well. She had a little boy and there were no problems. Not even any stitches. We brought her back into the labour room and I was making her a cup of tea. Then, when I went into the room with the cup of tea, she was shaking all over the place. I rang the bell for Sister. It was so scary and then she shouted for me to ring Doctor McKenzie and get him back."

I was trying to keep up with what Betty was saying. She was talking so fast and seemed stressed as she was telling me the events of the night.

"It has just been terrible. We have put her in the big double room on the right, the first room down from the office next to the bathroom. Doctor McKenzie is still in the room now and has been ringing doctors in Palmerston North since it happened and trying to decide whether to transfer her out or not. Not sure what they are going to do with her, as she is still unconscious and not out of the woods yet."

"What do you think I should do then?" I asked.

"I think just look after the other postnatal women and babies at the moment. Yes, just do that for now. They are getting a sister from Masterton to special Mrs Morris. Someone has to be in the room at all times. Don't worry, it will be the one of the sisters who will special her, so just concentrate on the other mothers and babies," Betty went on.

"You just have to be quiet. We're not allowed to make a sound. Smithy is going to have to put towels on all the trolleys so there is no noise. Look, I have to go and see what else there is to do because Sister is still in there with Doctor McKenzie. I have been absolutely frantic and have had to do all the feeds on my own, as well as everything else while all this has been going on."

"I just have to give you a quick handover so you can look after the ward and the nursery. You were here yesterday afternoon so at least you know the women. Mrs Butler had her baby early yesterday morning so I have done her last perineal swab and she'll have to be got up for a shower this morning. Her baby is starting to go on the breast, but she needs help with that. Mrs Evans is having oil packs for her engorged breasts. She is managing her baby independently, but the baby will need a weigh and also test weighing before and after feeds. Mrs Bates was keen to go home today so you will need to check her feeding. Baby will need to be weighed and Plunket will have to be notified for the postnatal follow up for her and baby. Just talk to her and make sure she will be able to manage baby at home and what support she has, as she is a primip. Check that she is happy and has no concerns. Then there is Mrs Morris's baby. He is being bottle fed at the moment in the nursery while Mum is so sick, but when Mr Morris comes back, he might like to have some time with the baby at some point. I think that is all at the moment. I had better get back to the room and see if there is anything else they want."

With that, she left the kitchen and closed the door behind her. Smithy had also just got to work and came into the kitchen preparing the trays for breakfast. I told her as much as I knew and that all the trolleys were going to have to have tea towels put on them to cut back any noise.

"Golly, that's awful," she said as she started to put the tea towels on the trolleys and prepare the trays for breakfast. Smithy was so dedicated to her job and thorough with everything she did.

I opened the door and went into the corridor. I didn't quite know what to do, but thought I had better find out. Gingerly I walked towards the double room where I knew Mrs Morris was and peered in. Doctor McKenzie was standing at the foot of the bed and I had never seen a more worried looking man. There was the drug trolley and another trolley with all kinds of equipment on it near the end of the bed where Mrs Morris lay. Sister Drury was standing at the side of the bed, looking exhausted after being up all night. Sister Foster appeared behind me as she obviously had realised something was going on in the room. She was on for the morning shift as well.

A look of shock came over her face as she peered into the room and saw Mrs Morris lying in the bed unconscious.

"We'll go into the office," said Sister Drury. "Can you just watch her for a bit, Nurse, while we go and talk?" she asked Betty. The three of them left and Betty and I just stood there. Betty made her way over to Mrs Morris's side.

"We are disturbing her as little as possible, so will hold off expressing any milk from her till she's conscious. Mr Morris has left to sort some things out at home, but will be back soon. He is so worried – it's all a nightmare for him."

"I might go and sort out the theatre and put it back together while you are still here. At least I can do that," I said.

"Well, Sister Foster will be in here till the Masterton midwife comes, so you will have to just carry on with everything else. Thankfully, I'm off tonight. I couldn't cope with another night like this one. I'm going as soon as Sister gets back," Betty said.

"Ok well, have a good sleep then," I said as I left. I started to think as I cleaned and put theatre back together.

'I must ask Sister what this eclampsia is and what causes them to fit,' I pondered to myself. I continued putting the theatre back in order, knowing that it would be one less task to do during the morning and it was better to be ready in case someone else came in – heaven forbid.

As I went in and out of the room, I saw Smithy putting the breakfast trays out on the covered trolley and Sister Foster talking to her. There was one trolley for the breakfast trays and another trolley for the cups of tea and coffee that would be taken out once all the women had their breakfast.

'It is going to be hard until this Masterton midwife comes,' I thought. 'I'll just have to go and ask Sister if there is something I'm not sure about, although hopefully I'll manage.'

All these thoughts were going on in my mind. I never thought anything like this could happen when having a baby. It never occurred to me that sometimes things could go wrong.

I had just finished cleaning the theatre and was about to go down to see the postnatal women, when the bell rang from the room where Mrs Morris was. I went to answer it. Sister Foster was in there and had rung the bell. She wanted me to watch Mrs Morris while she went to the toilet.

"Can you just stay here while I go to the toilet and ring the bell if she starts fitting," she said and off she went.

Mrs Morris was lying on her side and appeared to be in a deep sleep. I sat down beside her and just watched. She was breathing quite deeply and seemed to be so peaceful, like she was in a deep sleep. She looked so young with her small frame and shoulder length brown hair. After about five minutes I could see her body start to twitch and then start to shake a little. I just stood watching, wondering whether to ring the bell or not, as I watched her starting to shake and twitch.

'Is it getting worse?' In sheer panic I rang the bell. Not knowing if I should or not, but not feeling very happy about being in the room with her by myself.

Sister Foster quickly appeared in the room looking a little out of breath and flustered. She obviously felt I had rung for her unnecessarily and looked a bit miffed, as Mrs Morris had settled down again.

"Just ring me if she starts really shaking," she said and then sat down and I was free to go. I was relieved to leave the room.

I went into the milk room to make up the Karilac and the formula for the day. All that I needed to do for the nine o'clock feed ran through my mind. I went and got everything ready for bath time, getting all the linen out for the babies and setting up the baths. Then I went down to the mothers to see if they were ready to come to the nursery. Mrs Butler was keen to get out of bed and come down to see her baby bathed. One by one, they made their way down. I bathed Baby Butler while the other mothers got on with bathing their babies. They were all very aware of needing to do as much as they could to help out. When they had gone, I looked at the new baby whose mother was so very ill.

'You know nothing of what's going on do you, little one,' I thought as I started to change his nappies.

He was such a lovely baby, so small and precious. He looked around with his eyes wide open and eagerly took the Karilac as I put the bottle in his mouth. It was lovely to just have some time to sit down. It seemed like I'd been running since I'd arrived and it was lovely to give this baby some loving care that his mother couldn't give.

The midwife from Masterton arrived about mid-morning and Sister Foster was free to come out of the room.

"Would you like to go to morning tea now?" she asked.

I jumped at the chance of escaping the stressful atmosphere of maternity. The hospital was buzzing with what had happened and the other nurses from general kept prodding me for information. I tried to act a bit dumb, saying I didn't know much, but I was amazed how much they did know and how word had got around so quickly. Mrs Brunton, the matron, had come down to see what was going on before morning tea and obviously conservations had been overheard. A small hospital is like a small town. Everyone seems to know everything that's going on.

There were many meetings in the office during the morning with the sister, the doctor and the matron discussing the case and many phone calls to specialists in the bigger hospitals that were either 40 minutes or an hour away. It was decided not to transfer her to either of the bigger hospitals. I wasn't sure why, but probably the movement of an ambulance would make the journey too risky. It had been stressed that we weren't to make any noise and were to be as gentle as possible when moving her.

The morning continued to be busy. I helped change Mrs Morris's pad at regular intervals and helped give her a sponge bath. Having a midwife specialling Mrs Morris had taken the pressure off, leaving Sister Foster and I to look after the other women and do our normal work. Sister Foster was able to go into the office and do the paperwork that always seemed to take so much of her time.

I then took Mrs Butler down for her shower and showed her everything that was involved with that. There was a routine that we had to show every woman when they first got up for their shower. I had so much to do, but I knew I had to explain how to keep the perineum clean after showering and going to the toilet, even though I was sure a simple explanation would have done.

"Now when you have finished going to the toilet, Mrs Butler, you take this pack here, which has a pad in it and four sterile disposable towels. The pad you have taken off needs to go in this paper bag and be put in the rubbish. The first pad of the day needs to be put in the dirty utility room on the bench, so the sister can look at it. You need to write your name on it with the pencil that's there."

"Now use one of the towels and put it between your legs when going to the shower from the toilet. You then take it out and put it in the outside wrapping. Don't put it near the remaining clean towels or the clean pad. When you have had a shower, use the remaining towels to dry your perineum before putting on the clean pad. The dirty towels are then wrapped and put in the rubbish. Wrap them in the outside wrapping and put them in the bin. Here is a towel and flannel to use. I'll just put them here on this bench."

"I'll leave you to carry on. I won't be far away. Ring me by pulling on this cord if you need me or when you've finished. Definitely ring me if you feel faint. I won't be far away."

After Mrs Butler had finished her shower, it was nearly lunch time. The day was flying by.

There was tension in the air throughout maternity and everyone seemed stressed. The other women kept asking how Mrs Morris was and it was hard to know how to answer, since we weren't allowed to say anything about it.

She was still unconscious by the time I went off the morning shift, but had started to wake when I went to work the next morning. She was still very drowsy and needed a lot of rest and sleep. The Masterton midwife stayed and helped for about three days and spent her shifts specialling Mrs Morris, alternating with the other sisters.

When she had fully regained consciousness, we took the baby into Mrs Morris, just to be by her side to start with, then to have holds and to gradually introduce breastfeeding. We started by hand expressing the milk first and giving the milk to the baby. Then when she was up to it, she started breastfeeding.

Finally, after nearly a week, she started to care for the baby herself. It was a gradual and slow recovery and we were careful not to put too much stress on a woman who had been through so much. Day by day, Mrs Morris continued to slowly improve with no lasting ill effects. We spent a lot of time helping her and guiding her to care for her baby and herself.

Mrs Morris had pre-eclampsia, but because it was not diagnosed antenatally, she ended up having eclampsia with convulsions, a symptom of late stages of the disease. It was called the disease of pregnancy and if left untreated, could have devastating results for both mother and baby, as it nearly did for Mrs Morris and her baby.

It can come on very suddenly and can progress very quickly, as was the case with Mrs Morris. Fortunately, the baby was born before Mrs Morris started having convulsions. Otherwise, mother and baby could have been at risk of dying. It was fortunate, too, that the labour had been relatively quick and normal.

I can recall only one other case of eclampsia when I was working at the maternity annexe in the 1970s. It was a woman who was having twins and had been admitted for bed rest, as was the normal treatment when pre-eclampsia was diagnosed.

It was decided that she would be transferred to Masterton for the delivery of the twins, which was another risk factor that she had. She did go on to develop eclampsia while in Masterton Hospital and the twins were delivered by caesarean section. It was very fortunate that she had been transferred when she was, but unfortunate that she had not delivered prior to having the convulsions.

When the twins were about a week old and her condition was more stable, she was transferred back to us for mother craft skills and support to make sure she was able to care for the babies before going home.

Doctor McKenzie unfortunately died suddenly, not long after Mrs Morris had her baby and I often wondered if the stress of that night had contributed to his early death. Certainly he was missed in the town and mourned by all his patients and all who knew him.

Working in maternity, there were a lot of unexpected events. The women never had ultrasound scans antenatally, so unless picked up by palpation, complications occurred unexpectedly. There were cases of undiagnosed presentations, like breech babies (bottom or legs coming first instead of the head) and twins. There were also cases of babies being born that were malformed or had unexpected defects. Some of these babies were sent to the bigger neighbouring hospitals, while some babies were born with little chance of survival and died within hours of birth.

Little did I know that pre-eclampsia was going to have a

devastating effect on my own life that would impact me for years. I had no idea how this disease could cause such havoc in a woman's life, but I would find out in time.

Pink Magnolias

THE VIEW FROM THE STAFF kitchen in maternity was one of a beautiful, big magnolia tree that took over the entire area outside the window. Just beyond the tree was a path leading to a door, which opened to the corridor that linked the dining room and the maternity annexe. Looking out of the kitchen window, you could see people coming for appointments to the x-ray and physiotherapy departments. People used to make appointments if they needed an x-ray and Mrs Griffiths would take the x-rays during the day, between doing the administration work in the main office.

The magnolia tree had exploded into colour and it was a mass of flowers. They were the loveliest of flowers, shaped like a trumpet and the most delicate shade of pink, with a darker shade of pink at the base. Rex, Mrs Brunton's husband, was the gardener and he took great pride in keeping the grounds immaculate. The lawns were mown to perfection and the rose gardens dared not show a weed. When the roses came out, the hospital looked so picturesque. This spoke not only to the care of the gardens, but also to the care that the hospital gave. It was a community of caring individuals and everyone took pride in their place of work, which to many was more like a home, rather than just a place to come and earn money.

Sister McLaren started working at the maternity annexe a few months after I started. She was a midwife who had come from a small rural community an hour east of Pahiatua. The maternity annexe at Pongaroa had closed. In time, so did the other small maternity annexes around the area, including Woodville and Eketahuna. Pahiatua was the only maternity unit between Masterton and Palmerston North after the other maternity units closed. The sisters who were in charge of the closed maternity units came and worked at the maternity annexe in Pahiatua.

Sister McLaren had come from Pongaroa, Sister Shannon and Sister Southgate from Woodville, and Sister McDonald from Eketahuna. They were all older women who had been midwives for years and had worked for a long time in their communities. Sister McDonald had no family and she came and lived in the nurses' home. Sister Shannon was a widow with adult children and commuted from Woodville to work. Sister Southgate was married, with two teenage boys and also lived in Woodville. Sister McLaren moved to Pahiatua with her husband, Jack, and while Jack manned the bar at the Returned Services Association (RSA), Sister McLaren came to work at the annexe.

They all used to take turns at being on call for the night shift, although Sister Shannon began doing permanent nights soon after she started, much to the dismay of Betty who had her hours cut. This caused much friction between Sister Shannon and Betty, even though they never saw each other. I used to hear it from both sides, but mainly from Betty, making it even harder to get off duty on time when she came on. She was so angry about it all and felt it was very unjust that her job was being threatened. Sister Shannon was a very capable midwife and coped on her own with births during the night. She would call the doctor for a birth, but otherwise she just managed with whatever came through the door, no matter how many women and babies were already in.

One morning, Sister McLaren and I came on shift and a woman had been admitted during the night and was well established in labour. She was having her first baby and, at first glance, I thought that Mrs Stone looked awfully big and her stomach seemed to be a lot larger than I had seen before. Sister McLaren had disappeared over to the general side to see Mrs Brunton and I went in to see Mrs Stone. She was walking around the labour room, which I hadn't seen before as most women lay in bed while in labour.

"Let me know if you want me to rub your back," I said as I stood there, wanting to be of some use.

"That would be nice," she said as she turned her back for me to rub. She then started breathing heavily and put her hands on the top of her thighs.

"They are getting stronger," she said. I timed this one and it lasted a minute.

I had been at a few births now and when the contractions got to a minute long and were around five minutes apart or less, they seemed to be in good labour and progressing. As the contraction eased, she gradually stood up again.

"It is getting hard," she panted.

"Here's some water," I said, handing her the glass sitting on the locker. "I'll go and get you a fresh jug of iced water as this is a bit warm. Be back in a tick." I quickly went out to the kitchen to get some ice and fill the jug up.

Smithy was just about to give out the morning tea. She had the tray all set up with the two teapots, one for the tea and one for the water, as well as sugar and milk. I spied some sultana scones laden with butter on a plate as she was about to leave.

"Looks like lovely sultana scones for morning tea, Smithy. They're my absolute favourite. Hope I get down to the dining room to try one."

"Yes, Mrs Lewer made them. She is such a good cook," she said as she finished loading up the trolley.

Smithy headed out the door as Sister McLaren came back.

"How is Mrs Stone?" she asked as she came in the kitchen.

"Well they are getting stronger and lasting a minute now, probably two or three every ten minutes," I replied.

"Ok, well you had better get to morning tea while you can and I'll go and see her."

I took the jug of water into the labour room before going to the dining room, pleased that I was able to get a break. I grabbed a drink and scone and went outside with the other nurses from general. I was getting to know them all a bit better now. It was nice going outside – the weather was warming up and it was so lovely sitting outside in the garden.

"How is it in maternity?" Linda asked. "I hear you've got someone in labour."

I could never work out how they knew everything that went on in maternity, but they did. I suppose the kitchen staff knew and word just got around the hospital. Word travelled fast, that's for sure.

"All's going well," I replied.

"We've got theatre today, so it's busy. Most will go home later though, but it's busy this morning," said Linda.

I never envied the general girls on theatre day, as they had to look after all their patients plus the extra ones that came in for day surgery. Once again, I was grateful to be working in maternity.

'What a great job I've got. I'm so fortunate,' I thought to myself.

Back in maternity, things seemed to be heating up for Mrs Stone. I heard her from the doorway as I entered. The heavy breathing started as another contraction came and with the intensity of the pain she started to cry out. Silence again and a break for about a minute or so, then another contraction. I walked into the labour room and Mrs Stone was still standing, now at the side of the bed, leaning on the bed for support. Beads of sweat were all over her forehead and she looked red faced and hot. In between the contractions Mrs Stone was relaxed. She showed such strength and courage.

She was called an elderly primigravida and even though she had not yet reached her 30th birthday, she was considered old to be having her first baby. Mrs Stone told me later that she married when she was 28 and that everyone had thought that she was on the shelf and would never get married.

The determination was there that she was going to have her baby without pain relief and that she was going to tough it out. There was such an acceptance of labour and an endurance and strength in her.

"Would you get a cold, wet flannel, Nurse, and wipe her face. It won't be too long now, I'm sure. The contractions are really intense," said Sister McLaren as I walked into the room.

I went and wet a flannel and wiped Mrs Stone's face. She was so hot and you could feel the heat through the flannel.

"Thanks. Please can I have some water?" she asked.

I handed her the glass of water and took it from her as another contraction began. We stayed with her as the contractions kept coming, unrelentingly and unabated. As they kept coming, Sister and I supported her and held her up as I rubbed her back and Sister McLaren gave words of encouragement. Her husband was around, coming in and out looking like a lost puppy and probably feeling like one. He stood and observed, looking lost and not knowing quite what to do.

It was nearing lunchtime when the contractions started to change and Mrs Stone started to make the familiar pushing and grunting sounds of second stage.

"Mrs Stone, are you able to get on the bed now? I need to examine you and hear the baby's heartbeat again. It is a bit awkward in this position," asked Sister.

Mrs Stone lay on the bed after the next contraction. Sister McLaren got the pinard and firmly pressed the instrument on the lower abdomen.

"Yes, sounds fine. Now can you lie on your side while I examine how far on you are?"

Sister went and got a glove and put some gel on it. "Just tell me when you're ready, after the next contraction has finished."

The next contraction seemed to take ages to come, but after it had finished, Mrs Stone rolled on her side. Sister McLaren put her right index finger up Mrs Stone's back passage.

"Pretty sure you are fully dilated now, so we'll go into the theatre next door. Nurse, get the door as I pull the bed out."

With that, Sister took off her gloves, covered Mrs Stone and pulled the bed back. I quickly opened the door that led into theatre.

We wheeled her in and then got her to move onto the narrow theatre bed. I took the bed back into the labour room and met Mr Stone, who looked bewildered and worried.

"Won't be long now," I said. "There is a chair there for you. We'll come and let you know when the baby is born," I said, pointing to the chair at the end of the room.

I always thought it must have been so hard for the fathers-to-be, just being left in the labour room, able to hear what was going on, but not able to be part of the birth. Hearing their wives cry out in pain and feeling like a spare part to all that was going on. It must have been distressing hearing it all. Only when they heard the baby cry, was there any sense of relief.

By the late 1970s, though, the fathers-to-be were allowed into the delivery room to support their wives and partners when they were giving birth. They had to be gowned up and have a mask on and their shoes covered. It was almost treated like a sacred place or sanctuary. The husband had to be at the head of the bed and not down the other end, where it was all going on and he might see something or get in the way. No, he was there purely to support his wife, comfort her and be there at this special time. He was not allowed to take a peek at the private area, which only the privileged were allowed to see.

On the other side of the labour room door, Sister and I donned our white gowns, hats to cover our hair and masks. Mrs Stone was on the theatre bed. It was normal for primigravida women to push for two hours in second stage – that is, from being fully dilated to actually pushing the baby out. We waited until the head was seen at the entrance of the vagina before ringing the doctor, unless there were concerns. The doctors had busy practices so one of the skills of midwifery was getting the timing right. Call them too early and you would be wasting the doctor's precious time, ring too late and he would miss the birth, which between the two was the better option.

Mrs Stone was lying on her side and, with each contraction, I would lift the leg up high so that Sister could see what was happening and whether the baby was coming down.

"How much longer?" Mrs Stone asked as another contraction came to an end.

She was so hot and exhausted. I had a wet, cold flannel at the ready and wiped her sweaty brow after nearly every contraction.

"You are in second stage now, Mrs Stone, and you are doing so well. We can see your perineum bulging, so the baby is not far away. You are doing great. Just keep pushing with every contraction," Sister McLaren said, trying to encourage her not to give up.

Another contraction came and I saw the stomach harden and rise up. Mrs Stone breathed for a bit and then pushed down as if she was doing a bowel motion.

"Just push as hard as you can. We can see you're making progress. Just keep pushing while the contraction is still there. Make the most of it. Take another big breath and push as hard as you can," Sister McLaren kept telling her with every contraction.

Mrs Stone was a natural. She was so calm and controlled. With every contraction she followed her body and did what came naturally. I took my cue from her face and lifted her leg as each contraction came.

Now and then she would ask, "Can you see anything yet? Can you see the baby yet?"

After about an hour, we were starting to see the vagina open up.

Just a slight opening of the vagina at first and then slowly, with each push, a little more of the head could be seen.

"You are doing so well," I said to her. "We can see the baby slowly coming now." This seemed to give her more encouragement and she continued to push so well.

Sister McLaren had got out the delivery pack and had the trolley laid out, with all the linen along the back, the bowls on one side and the instruments lined up along the front. There was warm Savlon in one of the stainless steel bowls, white obstetric cream in the other and cotton wool balls in the larger bowl. It looked as if we were set up to do an operation as we stood there with all our regalia on – white gowns, masks and theatre hats.

As I lifted the leg again, the baby's head descended more and now a good amount of the head was pushing through on the perineum. Its dark, wet hair was now clearly visible.

"Call Doctor Symes now, could you Nurse. At this time of day I would say that he will be at his surgery. He is expecting a call."

With that, I went out the double doors to the phone. I gave a message to the receptionist that Doctor Symes was needed in maternity. The surgery was near the hospital grounds, so it didn't take too long for him to get over to us. The familiar banging of the door, clearing of the throat and sound of him putting on gumboots and apron soon followed. In he came, a big man with dark, wavy hair and thick, black-rimmed glasses.

"How is she going, Sister?" he asked.

"Good, very good, we can see a good amount of head now, so it shouldn't be too long," Sister replied.

Sister took the pinard and got Mrs Stone to roll on her back to hear the fetal heart. She pressed the pinard so hard that it looked as if she was pushing the baby through to the other side. She looked at her watch as she timed the beats per minute.

"Heartbeat is good and has been about 140 beats per minute for most of the labour."

Another contraction came and Mrs Stone pushed again. I held the leg up, which was getting rather heavy. Doctor Symes leaned over to Mrs Stone.

"Good, that is lovely, Sheila. Not long now. You are doing well and we can see the baby's head pushing through."

With that, he went over to the hand basin and started scrubbing up. The gloves and gown were on the trolley and he took a towel and dried his hands before putting the gown and gloves on.

"Could you do me up, Sister?" he said as he turned his back to Sister McLaren so she could do the gown up. He went to the foot of the bed, where I was holding her leg up. Then, with the next contraction, the baby's head was nearly crowning as it pushed through the perineum.

"You are nearly there, Sheila. Just keep pushing with each contraction. We will have the baby very soon," Doctor Symes continued.

I put the leg down for a rest. Her legs could hardly close now and I had to hold the leg up a little, even without a contraction, as the head was stopping her from closing her legs completely. I did hope this baby would come soon, as my arm was aching so much with constantly holding her leg up.

The head was now just sitting on the perineum and, with every contraction, the head eased a little more towards the light that was beaming onto the perineum. I did think that having a great spotlight shining on it as it took its first breath was more likely to put a baby off coming into the world, but light seemed to be deemed necessary.

I looked at Mrs Stone and, again, I could see the concentration come onto her face as she put her head down a bit and started to push again. I lifted the leg.

"That's right, just keep the pushes coming, nearly there," Doctor Symes said as he put his gloved hands on the baby's head. "Just pant, pant, it will be easy now. With the next contraction the baby will be born."

With that, another contraction and another push, the baby entered the world.

"There she is, a baby girl. Congratulations. Well done, Sheila." There was noticeable relief as the baby started to cry. There was always a sense of relief at any birth. It was the relief of the labour being over, the hard work being done and the baby being healthy and normal. What a joy. The baby was now crying on the bed as Sister cut the umbilical cord and started drying the baby. She wrapped the baby and handed her to Mrs Stone, who had just relaxed back and started smiling with pure joy.

"There you are, Mrs Stone, a beautiful little girl. You did so well." Sister said, handing the new baby to its mother. It was over, after all that effort and pain.

"Thank you everyone. Thank you so much." Mrs Stone took her baby and started looking at her with love in her eyes.

Attention now turned to the placenta as Doctor Symes started slowly pulling on the umbilical cord. The syntocinon had been given and now the placenta had to be delivered.

Mrs Stone started to look like she was in pain and seemed to be back in labour. She could hardly hold the baby as another contraction came.

"Take the baby, Nurse," Sister asked. The contraction seemed intense and Doctor Symes kept pulling on the cord to deliver the placenta.

"Sister, look, there is another bag of waters coming. Can you see that?" With that, a bulging bag of waters was at the entrance of the vagina.

"Get me an amnihook, Sister." Sister quickly handed an amnihook to the Doctor and he broke the bag of waters. Clear fluid came pouring out. We all stared as Mrs Stone started pushing again. Another baby was now on the perineum.

"We have another baby," Doctor Symes called as we all stared in disbelief. The baby was coming fast and Mrs Stone was pushing with all her might. The contraction seemed so strong. She didn't ask anything, she just pushed like she couldn't help it. The contractions were taking over her body again.

The baby was pushing the perineum open and was sitting there, waiting to be born with the next push.

"I just can't help it," Mrs Stone said as she pushed again and the head came out.

"You have another baby, Sheila," Doctor Symes called out as another baby was born with the next push.

"Another girl," he called. She cried like her sister.

"I don't believe it. Twins." Mrs Stone said. "Oh, oh no, twins. Is it two girls? I don't believe it, twin girls. How amazing!"

"Yes, well there are certainly two girls," Doctor Symes chuckled.

"We'll just deliver these placentas first and I'll go and tell Jim the good news."

With that, a placenta plopped out into the kidney dish followed by another placenta. We were all stunned as we all looked at the two girls that had just been born. I handed Mrs Stone the first twin and Sister gave her the other twin in her other arm. They were both so different. One had a long face and was blonde, while the other little girl had a round face and was a lot darker.

Doctor Symes took his gown and mask off and went out to give the news to the waiting father. He seemed to have a spring in his step and looked so pleased and relieved that all had gone so well. Sister and I quickly labelled the babies and dressed them so Mrs Stone could get out of the theatre.

"Well, that doesn't happen very often," commented Sister McLaren. "In fact, I have only had one other case in my midwifery career. It is such a surprise when it does happen."

We quickly gave Mrs Stone a sponge and put the abdominal binder on so we could take her out to her waiting husband. We decided to wheel her straight down to a double room, rather than take her back to the labour room. Grabbing Mr Stone, we wheeled the bed with Mrs Stone and her luggage down the corridor to her room.

"Are you still wanting to breastfeed?" Sister asked as we manoeuvred the bed into the room. "We've put you in a double room so you'll have plenty of room and privacy with the twins.

"Yes, I would really love to be able to feed them if I can," said Mrs Stone.

Mr Stone followed with a stunned look on his face that turned into a beaming smile when he was finally able to see his girls. We got the babies and gave them to their doting mum to see if they would go on her breasts. Sister and I put a baby under each of Mrs Stone's arms and helped attach them to the breasts, putting pillows under the babies for support.

"You're amazing," Mr Stone said.

We left them to spend time together and have a good look at the two beautiful lives they had made with each other. It was a time when we could relax the rules and give privacy to a couple who had a lot to plan and discuss. It was a shock to end up being parents to two babies when only one was expected.

News of the undiagnosed twins travelled like wildfire and, before long, maternity was inundated with phone calls enquiring about Mrs Stone and the twins as well as visitors trying to see her. At visiting times the room was so crowded. Even after visiting hours we had streams of people coming to the door wanting to come in and see Mrs Stone and her babies. It was strictly forbidden for visitors to come after hours, except husbands.

The visiting hours were from 2pm until 4pm so, of course, everyone came in those hours, meaning the room was packed. At 2:30pm, when we rang the nursery bell, there would be a flock of visitors to see the twins. The hour in the evening from 7-8pm was strictly for the husband to visit.

Mrs Stone was well-read on breastfeeding and was determined to breastfeed the twins. We gave her heaps of help and during most feed times we had the girls on either side of her, one under each arm and on each breast. It was lovely to see and eventually, as more milk came in, she was able to feed both the twins with ease, swapping sides each feed. The stay in hospital was longer than normal, as we gave support for the breastfeeding and helped with caring for the twins. We ensured all was well and that Mrs Stone could manage before she went home.

It was a delight to me when, in years to come, I was the midwife for one of the twins when she herself gave birth to her two children. We laughed when she told me that her mother was told to go on a diet because she was putting on too much weight when she was pregnant.

Head Over Heels

BARRY AND I HAD MET in 1968 during the summer break at the end of my second year of secondary school. I had previously seen him driving around town in his car with some mates and he had caught my eye. I didn't know him, but he had a cheeky smile and was very handsome with his blonde hair and blue eyes. He seemed to be the one that owned the car because he was always driving.

Marcia, my best friend from school, used to stay for weekends at times. We would walk up town to the milk bar and play the jukebox. We would often see him driving his light brown Ford Prefect around the squares in town with the window down and his elbow hanging out. He seemed to have a great time with his friends.

I couldn't believe it when I went to a New Year's Eve party that year and there he was with his mates. He looked over at me with a glint in his eye.

Was he interested in me? I observed him for an hour or two and during that time noticed he kept looking over at me and the group I was with. Halfway through the evening I decided what to do. With that, I leaned over to Janette, a friend I was with, and said, "Do you know that blonde guy in the jeans and light blue shirt?"

"Isn't his name Barry Watson?" she replied.

I turned and just blurted out, "Can you go over and say I am interested in going out with him?"

Janette didn't hesitate and off she went. I tried not to seem too obvious and looked around at what else was going on in the room. For me, if you wanted something, you needed to go after it. It was no use waiting for him to make the first move, as it might never have happened.

I was attracted to him in every way. I didn't know if he even knew my name, but I was willing to take a chance. He certainly was not at school, as I would have seen him there. No, he was working, had money and a car.

Next thing, back Janette came. "Yes, he's keen, and he is Barry Watson. I thought that was his name," she said. "He said to meet him outside in ten minutes".

Well, now what had I done? I was committed now and there was no backing out. It could have been awkward but it wasn't. He had had a few beers and I had a blackberry nip or two. We introduced ourselves and arranged to meet the following night, exchanging phone numbers and addresses.

"I've noticed you around for a while," he said. I felt a sense of satisfaction that I had not made a fool of myself and that he was as keen on me as I was on him.

Barry was working in a local garage doing his apprenticeship to become a motor mechanic and had two years to go. He was nineteen years old and I was fifteen. He was softly spoken, nicely dressed, casual and clean.

I was still at school and, as much as it had become rather boring for me, I knew that I needed to finish the next year. Mum and Dad had made that clear. I was alright with that though. Barry and I continued to see each other as much as we could, although mainly in the weekends. After the first date, we started phoning each other through the week and Barry would visit me at home sometimes in the evenings.

I had never heard of his family but when I mentioned them to my mother she knew Win and Lin, Barry's parents. She was happy for me. Their family was similar to ours and they had similar backgrounds. Both our families on both sides were from pioneering families who had come from Great Britain a few generations back.

"They are a very close family," Mum said. "Grandad knew Barry's grandfather. They were great mates and would often have a good old yarn when they met up town."

Well, no obstacles at all, even though I was only fifteen. We became very serious very quickly and, before long, we were spending all our spare time together. We would go out every weekend during the day and at night we would go to parties.

A lot of current bands used to come and play in the town hall and whenever they came, we would book our tickets and go. I loved music and knew every band and song that was at the top of the charts. It was at that time that Elvis's gold Cadillac came to town and was displayed in Ryan's Garage. Everyone was excited to go and see a car that Elvis had owned. It was great that it came to our small town as it toured New Zealand.

Marcia started going out with one of Barry's friends and would often come and stay. Barry always had a car, so we could go anywhere. Often we would go out with a group of his friends and mine. He had money and was generous with it, most of the time paying for petrol, smokes, meals and whatever we wanted. We would often buy beer and park up somewhere. There were a few favourite parking up spots around town and there would be others parked up as well. We all knew each other and if there was a party going on, word would get around and everyone would end up in the same place.

I loved fashion and would buy material from the local fabric shop in town. I would sew mini skirts and dresses mostly. That was the fashion of the day, thanks to Jean Shrimpton and Twiggy. The minis took so little material that you could sew one in less than a couple of hours. I was never allowed to buy clothes, but there were no limits when it came to buying patterns and material and making my own. Whenever I wanted clothes I would go to Fredricksen's, the local drapers, and buy the material and a pattern, booking it up to Mum's account. I had such fun sewing my own clothes and always had the latest fashion.

I even used to wear my school gym frock as short as I could. I would have the belt round my hips with the gym pulled up and hanging over the belt a little. Miss Price, the Head Mistress, used to go on about how long the gym frock should be, but she couldn't fight the fashion of the day. In the end she gave up, so long as we didn't wear them too short. My hair was thick, brown and long and I had a thick fringe cut in line with my eyebrows. I used to tease my hair up just past the fringe and then spray on hairspray to keep it in place. At school, hair was not allowed below the collar, so I mainly wore pig tails.

We weren't allowed to wear makeup at school, but when I went out I used to lay it on thick, especially around the eyes as was the fashion. I used to wear eyeshadow, eyeliner and mascara for the eyes and, for the lips, I mainly wore pale pink lipstick.

In the weekends we would sometimes drive to Palmerston North or one of the nearby beaches – Himitangi or Foxton beach. We would go in Barry's car or sometimes on his motorbike. We went through the Manawatu Gorge, zipping around the windy road and passing all the vehicles we could on the way. Wind in our faces, I would nestle behind Barry's back. On one side of the road were rock cliffs and on the other side a sheer drop down to the Manawatu River below.

Before long, Barry was coming out to the bach with us at Mataikona and was accepted as part of our family. We were inseparable during the following year and spent as much time as we could together.

By the time I had left school and started working at the hospital, Barry and I had been going out for over a year and he was very much part of our family. I had become very reliant and dependent on him for support. Whenever something went wrong or I was upset, I would ring him. He would fix it or talk it over with me and all would be well. He has always had such a strong sense of commitment and loyalty that I could rely on him no matter what.

It was inevitable that we would get engaged and get married. No one lived together then and most got married young. Barry asked me to marry him and I was so excited when we went and bought the ring at the local jewellers, Oxley's. It was a diamond ring with three stones across a yellow gold band, with the middle stone bigger than the two on the side. It was set in platinum and had a platinum scroll down either side. The ring cost $150 and Barry was earning $40 per week at the time.

We had an engagement party at our place. Dad was very good at organising and throwing parties. He was the perfect host and we had over 50 young people and relations crammed into our house. We got engaged in the year that I started working at the hospital and we were married in the following July.

I was seventeen and Barry was 21 when we got married on July 31st 1971. We were married in the local church where I used to go to Sunday school as a kid, like most kids did in the 1960s. Mum and Dad put on a beautiful, traditional wedding with 150 guests, mainly made up of Mum and Dad's friends.

Following the wedding and reception, everyone enjoyed live music and a dance with all the pop songs of the era – Elvis, the Beatles, Abba, the Rolling Stones, the Beach Boys and Herman's Hermits, to name a few. My bridesmaids were my sister, Lesley, and my best friend Marcia. Barry's five-year-old niece, Wendy, was my flower girl. The bridesmaids were dressed in purple gowns and carried mauve and purple bouquets. Wendy carried a lavender parasol with a frilly edge.

I had a white gown with a bodice covered in guipure lace and sleeves in the same lace. The gown was to the ground with a long train flowing behind that was attached to the waist at the back. The same lace that was on the bodice and sleeves was appliquéd onto the train like a cascade of tumbling flowers. We had a wonderful day and Barry and I were so happy. I had been working at the hospital for nineteen months when we got married. Sister Foster and Sister Drury came to the wedding and all the nurses that I worked with came as well – some to the wedding and some to the dance.

During the time of our engagement, we were at the bach with the family. It was one of the rare times that my grandmother was there.

"The Godfrey house is on the market. They only want six thousand dollars for it," she said.

"What, the one on the corner of Edward Street? The house down from your place?" I asked.

I loved that place and used to go past it whenever I visited my grandmother. It was full of character – a beautiful, big rough cast house with stained glass windows. We couldn't wait to get back to town and, first thing on Monday morning, we went and had a look at it. The house was beautiful and in its original condition. Nothing had ever been done to it since it was built in the 1930s. We put an offer in of five thousand dollars and our offer was accepted.

Grandad was a carpenter and offered to renovate the kitchen for us and, before we had even got married or moved in, he had transformed the kitchen and modernised it. The original coal-range oven was taken out and a modern electric stove put in. He used to wander down from his house to ours and just work away at his leisure. We would talk about how we wanted the kitchen to be and he would tell us what he needed for materials, then Barry would have it delivered. By the time we were married, it was all completed and we were ready to move in.

Born for Life

A Winter Honeymoon

AFTER SPENDING OUR WEDDING NIGHT at The Grand Hotel in Palmerston North, we travelled to Ohope Beach the next day. We booked a cabin at Ohope Beach for our honeymoon, not thinking of what the weather would be like in July. Arriving in the late afternoon, we got out of the car and looked at the little, wooden cabin on the beachfront facing the open sea.

It was a lot smaller than we had envisioned. We unpacked the car and explored the hideaway that was ours for the next week. There was a living room with a couch and table and chairs. The one bedroom was off the living room and had a double bed with a chest of drawers. At the other end of the living room was a small kitchen. The cabin was self contained with everything we needed.

We looked out the tiny windows from the bedroom to the view of the beach and sea beyond.

"Well, it'll be cosy," I said. "We have plenty of blankets, the linen is clean and fresh and there is a heater if it gets too cold."

"It's not exactly what I thought it would be. I thought it would be a bit more than this." Barry appeared to be disappointed in where we were staying.

"Look, come here," I said. We hugged each other and felt the warmth of our love for each other. "It'll be perfect. We'll be alone with no phone, no television, just you and me together all week and no one else."

"You're right. It's perfect. Our own little hideaway and it's very quaint," he agreed.

We started making it comfortable by making the bed, putting the heater on and unpacking the few food items we had brought. Before long it was warm and cosy. We climbed into bed as the rain started and we cuddled each other with the sound of rain on the tin roof drowning out any words we were saying. Words were not needed though, as we knew we loved one another. This was going to be our haven for the week. What bliss.

The little heater provided some warmth, but the greatest warmth was generated by our love for each other. It didn't matter when we got up, we had the whole day to waste and enjoy. What a great sound – rain pounding down on a tin roof – to snuggle up to and feel cosy and warm.

It rained every day that first week in August, but we didn't care. Between showers and when we were not in our cosy bed, we went for walks along the beach, rugged up in our warm jackets and scarves. It was cold and bleak as we walked along the wet, sandy beach. Out over the sea was a misty hue and the sea rolled in with the sound of crashing waves. We hugged each other as we walked, keeping close and warm at the same time.

We had the beach to ourselves all week and didn't see or speak to anyone else. I tried to impress Barry with my cooking skills and cooked breakfast every morning, along with cereal, fruit and, of course, coffee.

We booked the cabin, not realizing how perfect a winter holiday at the beach would be. No other holiday would have given us the solitude to just spend the time alone together. We were in our own world and no one else mattered.

After a week, we were ready for home and looking forward to setting up our house. When we got home, all the wedding presents were on the living room table and spread around the lounge room. Mum and Dad had dropped them in after the wedding dance, ready and waiting for our return. We spent the next few days finding places for all our gifts – some useful, some ornamental. People had been so wonderfully generous and kind that we virtually had all we needed for our home.

When each room was set up, we talked about how we were going to decorate it in the future. We made plans while we were home and had time to talk about what we were going to do to make the house more livable.

Mum and Dad and Barry's parents were frequent visitors, helping whenever they could and giving advice when we asked. Barry's parents supplied us with mutton and lamb from their farm from the time we were married until they got too old. They never asked for money for the meat, just a hand on the farm when needed. So every shearing or docking time, Barry was down on the farm helping and I would go and spend time with Barry's mum.

From the time I knew Barry, his mother never bought biscuits or cake. She baked every week and the tins were never empty. Morning and afternoon tea were always served on an embroidered tablecloth, the cake and biscuits were put out on china plates and the tea was made in a teapot.

There were very few flower beds when we moved into our house, so we started planning the gardens around the house. Dad had been a florist and a nurseryman, so gardening was in my genes. I loved gardening when I was growing up, so it was something that I wanted to do. The house was situated on a corner section and once the big, old marcracapa hedge was pulled down, the house was visible from both streets and very open. Barry set about laying new lawn and I planted two big rose gardens on the front lawn with flower beds right around the house. The house was a 1930s stucco bungalow with a huge veranda right around the front of the house and a door at each end of the veranda leading into the house. One led into the large lounge and the other into one of the bedrooms.

Barry and I had a week at home after our time at Ohope Beach. During that week, I visited the maternity annexe to find out what my shifts were for the coming weeks. Sister Foster greeted me with open arms and seemed thrilled that I was back and ready for work again. I was excited to get back to work and life was full of adventure, love and fun. We were so happy and looking forward to our new life. We both had good jobs and a house that we had bought, which we were planning to put our own stamp on. Barry and I started work on the Monday, him back at Barrett Motors and me back at the maternity annexe.

Back at Work

MY FIRST SHIFT BACK STARTED at 2:30pm. I was still using the car to go to work while Barry used the motorbike. I parked the car and walked up the familiar ramp to the main door of the annexe. I briefly stopped at the sisters' office to say "Hi" to Sister McLaren and Sister Foster on my way into the changing room. My cape and all my uniforms already had my name changed. It was not much of a change going from Watts to Watson.

I quickly changed and went into the kitchen.

"We can go to afternoon tea now," said Christine. I have already taken the sisters their cup of tea".

"Great, let's go then and you can tell me what has been going on since I've been away."

"It has been quiet over the past couple of weeks. Not many births at all. It has been quite boring, in actual fact. Anyway, how was the honeymoon? Did you have a good time and where did you end up going? We were all wondering, as you hadn't told anyone and there was no postcard," she asked.

"Well, we stayed at The Grand Hotel in Palmerston North for the first night and then spent a week at Ohope Beach in a little cabin. We couldn't have wished for a more amazing time and it was so peaceful.

The weather was terrible but we didn't care about that. We then spent last week at home sorting the house out. What a job, but nearly done. You will have to come around and see it now that we have moved in. Come around when we both have days off. I'll check the roster when we get back," I told her.

It was too cold to go outside so we sat with two of the general girls in the dining room for afternoon tea before heading back to maternity.

Everything seemed the same and it looked as if nothing had changed. Well, what can change in two weeks really? I checked the roster and since Christine and I were off the following Thursday, we made arrangements for her to come around home on the following Thursday morning.

I went and collected the tea tray from the sisters' office.

"Welcome back, Julie. Did you have a nice holiday even though the weather was freezing? Well, it was here at least," Sister McLaren asked.

Protocol was starting to ease a bit and I was now being called by my first name. I thought it might have been because I had got married, but I noticed the sisters started calling all the nurses by their first names. We still called them 'Sister.' That had not changed.

"We had a lovely time and even though it was cold we didn't notice it too much," I smiled as I said it and they knew what I meant.

Sister McLaren was on for the afternoon shift and since it was quiet with only two postnatal women in with their babies, it was nice to just spend some time talking with the women and not have any time pressure.

Both the women that were in were multigravidas. That is, they had had a baby before, so they were experienced mothers. They were in having a rest, as much as anything else, and needed little assistance from the staff. They were experienced breastfeeders and could care for their babies independently. Apart from checking that they were alright and if they needed anything, there was little to do for them. There was no pressure for them to go home and even though they didn't need a lot of help, they were still able to stay in for a week if they wanted to.

Very rarely did women go home early, maybe at three days, but on the whole it was accepted that women needed a break. They were encouraged to stay in where everything was done for them and they didn't have the pressure of running a home and looking after the family.

The first task of the afternoon shift, once the visitors had gone, was to take each woman's temperature and pulse and ask them if their bowels had moved, writing the recordings down in a notebook. I then went around checking what needed doing. The autoclaving and sterilising seemed to be all up to date and all the rooms were well stocked and there was nothing needed in them.

I went into the theatre room, labour room and 'prep' room. All was in order and everything looked clean, neat and tidy. Every room reminded me of a hotel room waiting for guests to arrive. All the beds were made with clean, crisp linen and the towels were hung up on the side of the lockers.

Walking back down the corridor, Sister McLaren was sitting at the desk in the office. She caught my eye.

"Tell me all about your holiday and where you went," she asked. I hesitated and then walked in and sat down in the chair by the desk.

It was as if Sister McLaren just wanted to talk and she seemed genuinely interested in where we went.

"I did ask your father down at the RSA where you had gone, but he didn't know. 'They didn't tell me anything,' he said."

I laughed. "Well we wanted to keep it to ourselves until we got back, but we did give them a ring from the phone box while we were there."

Throughout the shift, Sister McLaren and I chatted between doing what needed to be done and checking on the mothers and babies at intervals. Things were becoming more relaxed. I even felt like I could have got my knitting out and done it if I had thought to bring it.

It was a small maternity unit of twelve beds and there were many times when it was quiet. Trying to keep busy, or look as if you were busy when you weren't, was hard. Even though you could spend some time talking to the women, they didn't want you there all the time. I sensed that things were becoming more relaxed and barriers were breaking down. As long as the work was done, the sisters didn't mind us sitting in the office with them. We could spend time getting to know each other.

The sisters were all older women and since there was only me and a sister on duty for a lot of the shifts, I got to know them and became more relaxed around them as bonds grew. Always, though, knowing my place and never crossing the line. As long as I showed them respect and always deferred to them when decisions were made, we got on well.

Each sister had a different personality and different ways of doing things, so once you sorted that out, it seemed to work. I found it was better to say too little than too much and to always think before opening my mouth.

Baby for Adoption

IT WASN'T SOCIALLY ACCEPTABLE IN the early 1970s to have a baby if you weren't married, and if someone did get 'in the family way', the pregnancy and birth would be shrouded in secrecy, leading to a lot of gossip in the town if people did find out.

Most girls that got pregnant and weren't married disappeared for a few months to a home for single mothers. They would have their baby and then come back to town and carry on with their lives as if nothing had happened. Their babies would be adopted out to a couple and would never be seen again by the woman who had given birth to them.

We often had a baby in the nursery waiting to be adopted. The mother would give the baby a set of clothes or a soft toy as a gift. After that, she left the baby with us while the adoptive parents were being chosen by a social worker. The mother would often have delivered her baby out of town and the baby would come to us to await adoption by a couple. Sometimes the baby was with us for several weeks before all the paperwork was completed and the adoptive parents were chosen.

The adoptions were not open, so the mother was giving up all her rights to the baby and to be part of her baby's life. They never saw each other again, but it was believed that the mother was giving the baby a chance in life that it never would have if it was brought up by a single mother. It wasn't until the mid-1980s that birth parents and their children could legally find each other and adoptions were open.

Anna was five-and-a-half months pregnant when she turned up at the maternity office to book in to have her baby. She arrived with her mother soon after the medical centre rang to say she was coming over. I showed Anna and her mother into the office before getting Sister Southgate, who was on that morning.

I was going down the corridor to the kitchen when Sister appeared at the door.

"Anna is here, Sister. She is here with her mother. The one the medical centre rang about."

"Is she here already? Alright, Julie, I'll be at least an hour doing all the paperwork and then I'll be doing an assessment in the labour room, so if you could just look after the rest of the ward and call me if you need me. The medical centre said that this baby was going to be adopted out, so I'll be a while, as I need to contact the social worker and talk to her."

The medical centre had sent Anna over to maternity to book in to have her baby with us. Her mother was with her as Anna was living with her parents. Even though the parents had been shocked and disappointed that their sixteen-year-old daughter had become pregnant, they were standing by her. Anna could have gone to a Salvation Army home for pregnant girls to have her baby there, but since her parents were happy for her to be with them, she was staying in town.

I didn't see Anna again until the day she came into labour. She arrived with her mother when her waters broke and she started having contractions. The contractions were very mild and she had come in early, but rather than send her back home, Sister Drury prepped her and she stayed in the labour room. She appeared so frightened and anxious and I would go in and talk to her, hoping that some reassurance would help her feel calm. Her mother was supportive and stayed with her.

Anna hadn't attended any antenatal classes, as she had felt too ashamed to go, so she had no idea what to expect. She had no idea what was happening to her body and the pain seemed to cause her even more anxiety and fear. I went and got heat packs for her back. She had several baths and just walked around the labour room not saying a lot.

The pain seemed to be getting more intense and Anna was crying out more and more with every contraction. The contractions were still irregular and mild to moderate in strength, but every time they came, Anna would cry and call out. She was terrified.

Sister Drury was on duty and would come in and out at times to listen to the baby's heartbeat and see how Anna was coping. Near the end of the shift, Sister decided to examine Anna to see if she was progressing at all.

"Get me a pair of gloves, Nurse, and I'll see how she is going. You are doing well, Anna, but we'll just see if you are dilating inside."

Anna lay on the bed on her side and pulled her knees up as Sister put her gloved index finger up Anna's back passage. Anna cried out as the finger went in.

"Sorry, Anna, I have to do this to see if you are progressing and to see if this baby is coming," Sister said as she moved her finger around inside.

"You still have a long way to go," Sister said in a concerned tone. "You're about three centimetres dilated; the cervix is still quite thick and the head is high." Sister pulled her finger out and got Anna to sit up.

"I'll ring the Doctor and see if we can give you something to help you sleep and help with the pain. You're finding it hard so if we give you something now, it might help you relax overnight. Mum can sleep in a chair or she could go home and come back in the morning. You can talk it over with Mum, while I go and ring the Doctor."

Anna started crying. She seemed so distressed about what was happening, not knowing how long the pain was going to continue.

Sister came back with an injection of pethidine. Anna lay on her side as Sister gave her the needle. Her mother decided to stay, as Anna seemed too distressed for her to leave and probably would not have coped well if she had no one with her.

It was near the end of my shift and Anna had become more relaxed as the pethidine took effect. She stayed in bed and was dozing between contractions. I went into the room and said my goodbyes to Mrs Hyde, Anna's mother.

"I'll see you tomorrow," I said. "I'm going off now but will be back tomorrow afternoon. Say goodbye to Anna for me when she wakes again. Hopefully she will dilate overnight and have her baby now that she is relaxed. I'll see you tomorrow then."

Betty had arrived for the night shift and after Sister had given her a handover, I got dressed into my clothes and headed out the door. Sister Drury was on call overnight in the nurses' home and was on again the next afternoon with me.

I had a lovely sleep and woke the next morning to a quiet house. Barry had already gone to work and hadn't woken me. A nice sleep in was what I needed. I was getting used to full-time shift work.

With all that had happened in the last few months, I was tired. It had been a whirlwind time and we were still settling into our house and married life. I spent the morning tidying up, putting more presents in their places and moving things around.

When I got to work in the afternoon, Sister Drury was already in the office with Sister Southgate.

"You girls need to go down to the office and get your pay. Mrs Griffiths has just rung for you to go to the office and get it," Sister Drury called out as I was going past.

"Ok, I'll just get changed and we'll go."

I quickly got changed and came to see who the nurse aide was on for the morning. I found Marcia in the labour room with Anna.

I went in and told her what Sister had said and, with that, we made our way down the corridor to the main office. When we arrived, all the general girls were already there and we lined up behind them. It was Thursday and every second Thursday was payday, so we had to go down to Mrs Griffith's office and all line up to get our pay and sign for it.

Once we had signed the book, we received an envelope with our payslip and our pay in cash. We had to go when we were called by Mrs Griffiths and, if not, then we would have to come back when she was there, but sometimes with all her x-ray appointments it was hard catching her.

When we got back, we went into the labour room to see Anna. Both sisters were in there discussing what was happening. Marcia and I stood there listening. Anna was still having contractions and finding labour hard.

"Doctor Symes has been in on his way back from lunch and is coming back again after surgery finishes at 5:30pm," Sister Southgate said.

"Anna dozed for some of last night but, by the time we came on this morning, we had to give her more pethidine. She was about six centimetres then and not coping again. Doctor Symes came in at 8am before he went to the surgery and said to carry on if the heartbeat is ok. She probably needs another assessment now and then he will see what to do next when he comes in after surgery."

"Alright, I'll check her again when you go off. Has the heartbeat been good? Sister Drury asked.

"Heartbeat has been fine. You can hear it clearly down on the lower left hand side. Someone has to stay with her all the time to help her cope. Marcia has been in here all morning and it helps if someone is supporting her. Her Mum has been here as well," Sister Southgate said.

Both the sisters headed out the door. "Could you stay with Anna, Julie? I'll be back soon to examine her. Marcia, it's time you were off now. You haven't had afternoon tea, so you might as well go."

"Thanks, Sister." Marcia replied.

She turned to me and said in a soft voice. "It has been so hard this morning. I have been with Anna all shift and I'm not sure whether she is getting anywhere. She has been in and out of the bath and we have all been trying to encourage her.

Mrs Hyde has been wonderful rubbing her back and you can duck out now and then, so long as someone is with her. I'll catch up with you when we both have days off. I'll check the roster tomorrow and give you a ring."

"Ok, that will be nice. Have a nice day off tomorrow," I said as she walked out.

Sister Drury was back in the room – glove in hand – to check Anna's progress.

"Well, you are nearly there," she said as she was doing the examination. "You're about nine centimetres so you are progressing, Anna. Slowly, but you're getting there. Roll over and I'll listen to baby."

Sister took the pinard and pressed it onto Anna's abdomen. "Heartbeat is strong so we will continue till Doctor Symes arrives unless you want to push. So don't be discouraged. It shouldn't be too long now. I know you have had a long haul but it's nearly over."

Anna looked at both of us with a look that was mixed with exhaustion and despair. Mrs Hyde came around to the bed.

"Look how well you've done, Anna. I'm sure it won't be long now. Just listen to the nurses." With that, she handed Anna a glass of water to sip and started to sit her up.

I stayed with Anna as Sister Drury popped in and out between looking after the rest of the women who were in the annexe.

There were two mothers in. They were a few days postnatal and had both had babies before, so they could look after their babies without much help. Because we had been so busy with Anna over the past 24 hours, the women were coming down to the nursery at feed times to get their babies and then taking them back to the nursery after feeding them.

Sister also had paperwork to do. There always seemed to be a lot of that, although I never knew what it entailed. After a birth, the paperwork would take over two hours, while the nurse aides did all the cleaning up, helped the women with the initial breastfeed and made the couple a cup of tea and toast. It was all part of our duties. Not that I minded it. I loved it and enjoyed being part of a family's special time. Sister would always come and check on the blood loss and blood pressure to see if all was well, but we did the more hands-on work.

Anna started showing signs that she might be ready to push. She had started grunting and the pattern of the contractions had changed. I went and got Sister.

"I think we'll move Anna into theatre now. Doctor will be here shortly and it sounds as if she's fully dilated. We'll let her push if she wants to and then Doctor can do an assessment when he comes. There's no point in me doing one as well."

For the next hour or so, we encouraged Anna to push with all her might. Sister and I were both yelling at her to push and Anna was faithfully putting her trust in us. Her face was red with all her efforts and perspiration was beaded all over her forehead. Cold flannels were flopped on her face and around her neck between contractions.

Doctor Symes arrived after Anna had been pushing for over an hour. There was nothing to be seen and it seemed like all her efforts were in vain. I felt so sorry for her.

'All this work, effort and pain for her baby that she will never care for,' I thought. It was so unfair, after all that she had been through.

After Doctor Symes had finished examining Anna, a decision was made.

"We will have to move her to the main theatre, Sister. She is fully dilated and has been pushing well, but the baby is still fairly high. We are going to have to do a high forceps. I'll ring Doctor Urwin from

Eketahuna to do the anaesthetics, as she will have to go under for us to do it. I'll go and ring him now while you take her around."

Sister went next door to the labour room to let Mrs Hyde know what was happening. She came back.

"I'll ring general and see if they can spare a nurse just to be here while we're in theatre. We can't really leave the annexe unattended."

Sister rang over to general and, within minutes, someone had come over to be in maternity while we were round in theatre.

"Just come and get me if something happens. I'll be in the main theatre and here are the other sisters' phone numbers. They are not on call, but just in case I can't get back. Come to me first though," Sister explained to the nurse aide who had come over to man the fort. We wheeled the bed down the corridor to the main theatre and then got dressed in our theatre hats, gowns, masks and shoe covers.

We got Anna on the theatre bed and moved the other bed out the door. By the time we had set up the birth pack and got the forceps and table set up, Doctor Symes and Doctor Urwin were present. It seemed such a stark, sterile place with nothing on the walls but white paint and a clock. The anaesthetic machine was huge and intimidating. I had never been in the room before. If I had not had so much to do and my mind was not so occupied, I would have been overwhelmed.

Doctor Urwin was at the head of the bed with the anaesthetic machine. He calmly put the mask over Anna's face and, within minutes, she was not with us.

"Now, Sister, you and the nurse get on both sides of her and, when I tell you, both of you push from the top of her abdomen," Doctor Symes instructed.

Doctor Symes got out what looked like giant, steel salad servers and started putting white obstetric cream all over them. Sister and I got in position and I had to stand on a stool. The bed seemed so high.

Carefully, Doctor Symes put the forceps into Anna's vagina. They seemed to go so high up and the rod of the forceps was about halfway up inside her. He moved them around inside to get them in place over the baby's head.

"Sister, can you listen to the baby's heart before I start." With that, Sister Drury put the pinard to Anna's abdomen.

"It's all good, Doctor. Heart rate is about 130."

Doctor Symes was all gowned up and standing at the foot of the bed. He started pulling, gently at first. Eventually he was pulling as hard as he could and then he stopped. He took the episiotomy scissors and cut into the perineum. I looked down at the large flesh wound below where the forceps were.

"The baby feels as if it has moved down a bit. So Sister, I want you and Nurse to push on the top of her abdomen as I pull. We should get it."

All I could think of was Anna. She was not feeling what was happening and she had been spared any more pain.

Doctor Symes put one foot on the bed and pulled with all his might, pushing against the bed to get traction. Sister and I pushed from the top of the abdomen as hard as we could to push the baby down. As Doctor was pulling, he called out to Sister.

"When the head comes out, I want you to push down just above the pelvic bone in case the shoulders are a problem."

He just pulled and pulled. I just stared as the rods of the forceps started moving down. I was pushing as hard as I could on Anna's stomach, pushing her baby down to where it needed to come out. It seemed as if the baby's head would come off – the force that was being used was so great. Doctor Symes was pulling with all the force he could and slowly the baby seemed to be moving.

"One more pull and we'll have the head," he said as he rested for a minute between pulls.

With the next mighty pull, the head came out. Sister moved her hands down to press above the pelvis. The baby turned and the shoulders and body came out. The relief felt by everyone in the room was palpable. Doctor Symes smiled as he cut the cord and passed the baby over to Doctor Urwin.

"Thanks, Ken," he said as the baby was handed over.

Doctor Urwin put the baby on the table next to him and Sister went over to help. The baby came out stunned, limp and blue. He had two large, red marks on both checks of his face from the forceps. Doctor Urwin put a mask over the baby's head and started giving him oxygen. Sister rubbed the baby with a towel and dried him down. It seemed an eternity before there was a weak cry and he started to change colour to the lovely pink that I was used to. It was a few more minutes before the cry became stronger.

Doctor Symes asked me to give the injection for the placenta to come and, before long, it had plopped out.

We were all relieved that the baby, when it finally arrived, was healthy. The baby was a boy, weighing eight pounds, which was big, especially as it was her first baby.

Anna never saw her baby. We called him Jimmy and took him to the nursery and kept him in a cot down the back, so the public couldn't see him when they came to see the other babies. Mrs Hyde wanted to see the baby before she took Anna home two days later. Doctor felt it was better that she go home as soon as she could and see him in the surgery if she needed to. An injection was given to dry her milk.

On the day she left, she gave us a set of clothes and a small stuffed teddy for the baby to have. She was discouraged from seeing the baby but I don't know if anyone really talked to her about it. It was as if she just had to leave and get on with her life. As she left that day, she came down the corridor and left the clothes and toy in the office. Both the baby's mother and grandmother looked downcast and sad.

"I'm sure they will find a lovely home for your baby. You're doing the right thing. Remember that you are giving your baby a chance for a better life," Sister said, trying to comfort and reassure them that what was happening was for the best. They nodded, not that convincingly, and walked out the main door of maternity.

Night Shift

SISTER SHANNON WAS DUE TO go on a week's holiday and Sister Foster asked if I could work her nights while she was away.

I had done nights before but not that often, as there were two permanent staff that did all the nights. Betty worked two shifts a week and Sister Shannon worked five shifts. The other sisters took turns at being on call when Betty was on. They spent those nights in the nurses' home in case they were needed in the night. Once Sister Shannon started working at Pahiatua maternity annexe after Woodville maternity annexe closed, the other sisters only had to be on call when Betty was on nights.

I arrived at 10:45pm for the first of my five shifts. It was dark and cold as I left home for work. I was sure it would be a frost in the morning, so I covered the car windscreen with an old sheet, before going up the ramp to the main door of the annexe and into the office.

'Most people would be tucked up in their nice warm beds,' I thought.

Sister Southgate was in the office when I walked in. She was waiting for me to arrive and was all packed up and ready to go.

"I am on call tonight. I am in the first room on the left as you go in, right next door to the lounge," she said. "All is calm at the moment and we've had a good shift. I sent Debbie home about ten minutes ago, since she's on in the morning."

She then gave me a report on the mothers and babies that were in. Mrs White was having breastfeeding issues and had a breast binder on, which would need heating in the night after feed time. The baby was having test weighs before and after feed times. It was her first baby and she needed help with breastfeeding to latch the baby to the breast. There was Mrs Lund who was managing her baby well. It was her second baby and she shouldn't need any help. She wanted to go home in the morning.

Then there was Mrs Aitken, who had her baby earlier in the day and was still having perineal swabs. She had not long had one and since it was night, she could have the next one early in the morning. It was her first baby as well.

"Alright, Sister. Hopefully you will get a good night's sleep and I won't have to call you."

I walked down the corridor with Sister to the door that led to the nurses' home. I locked the door behind her as she walked through the covered passageway.

It was eerie and silent as I made my way back along the corridor. Getting a torch from the office, I made my way around the ward, checking that the doors were all locked and secure. It was so quiet. The only lights that were on were the night lights that were at intervals along the length of the corridor. As I made my way back down the corridor, I went into the rooms where the women were. Mrs White and Mrs Lund were in the double room at the far end. Peering in to see if they were alright, I heard the loud breathing noises of Mrs Lund. Obviously sound asleep. Mrs White was opposite and lying wide awake.

"Are you alright? Can I get you anything?" I said shining the torch into her bed space.

"Can I have some pain relief? My breasts are so sore and I just can't sleep," she said as she started to sit up.

"Ok. I'll go and get you some paracetamol. I won't be a moment," I said as I made my way to the office where all the drugs were kept behind the door. I was able to give out the drugs in the cupboard if they were charted, but wasn't allowed into the controlled drug cabinet, which was locked. The sister always had the key for that cupboard. I took Mrs White the tablets and some water before going to the next room where Mrs Aitken was. She was still awake, but when I asked her, she said she was fine and just trying to get to sleep before the next feed time.

I came down the corridor and went into the nursery where the three babies were sleeping.

'That's good. They're all asleep,' I thought. I saw all the bundles of nappies that needed folding and putting away, as well as Vaseline squares to fold.

'I'll do that soon. It's first things first. A cup of tea is in order.'

I came back into the office, cuppa in hand, and started reading all the notes.

'Well, that's it. There is nothing else, just what Sister told me,' I thought, as I finished reading the notes.

I sat down and looked at the clock. A quarter past eleven. It was going to be a long night. Eight hours seemed an eternity away. How could I stay awake and keep myself occupied for all that time? Fortunately I had brought some knitting for the wee hours of the morning – a lumber jacket I was knitting Barry.

I got up, went into the nursery and started folding the nappies and stocking up the cots with the linen needed for the next day. As I went out the door to go to the linen room, I was startled by a figure coming from the door that led to general.

"It's only me, Julie. Just thought I would come over and check you were surviving over here." It was Jenny, a nurse from the general side.

"Whew, you gave me a turn, a heart attack actually. It will take me all night to calm down again. Thanks for coming over though," I said.

We made our way into the office and started to chat. Jen was on permanent nights and was used to them. She talked ever so loud as if it was the middle of the day, not the dead of night when everyone should be sleeping. I closed the door slightly as she carried on. Even though she was loud, it was nice to have someone to chat to for a bit to help the night pass. It was also nice to know that there were others who weren't far away. If I needed them and phoned them, they would be here in a flash.

"Well, I'd better get back. We have a full ward at the moment and it's nearly time for the next round. I might see you later," she said as she started to open the door.

"Yes, come back when you can. It's just nice to know I'm not completely alone."

"Ring if you need anything and we'll be straight over. See you later," she said as she headed back.

I went back into the nursery to finish folding the linen and do the Vaseline squares. It was a monotonous job, but at least it was something to do. I then went to the prep room to see what needed doing. I restocked all the cupboards and made up some soap mix for the enemas.

'At least if I get all these jobs done, it'll be ok if someone happens to come in labour,' I thought to myself.

All the jobs that were done on nights really helped during the day. Everything was ready for the day, as all the restocking was usually done by the night staff. Satisfied that everything was done, I went back to the office and got out my knitting.

It was soon time for the one o'clock feed. I went into the milk room and got the Karilac and the containers ready so the women could clean their breasts. I then went into the nursery and started changing the babies. So far, they had all been fine. There was no crying and no need for them to be put in the dog box. I changed Baby White's nappy, put him on the scales and then took him out to his mum. I took the breast pads that she had on, brought them back and put them on the sterilizer to warm up. Her poor breasts were huge and looked so red and sore.

"Try and put him on the breast first and I'll be back soon. I'll just get the other babies out first," I said as I handed her little bundle to her.

I could see she would need a hand as her breasts were so engorged and full. The baby would find it hard to get a hold.

"Ok," she said. "I'll have a go. I haven't had a lot of joy so far though."

"I'll be as quick as I can. Perhaps try him under the arm this time. A change of position may help." With that, I quickly went back to the nursery.

I changed the other two babies and took them out. It would be alright to leave Mrs Lund, as she was an experienced breastfeeder. I picked up the bottle of Karilac for Baby Aitken and took the baby to its mother.

I rushed back to Mrs White when all the babies were out to see how she was doing.

"I get him on and then he just comes off. He just can't seem to stay there. He slides off after a few sucks." She looked so despondent, as if she had given up. The baby was put between her legs as she waited for me to come and give her a hand.

"I'll see if you can get him on. Might be best if I hold him in place for a bit and once your breast has some milk taken out, it will make it easier for him to keep going."

I stood there for nearly ten minutes trying to connect the baby with the breast. At last he started to suck. Once he got on and took some milk, he kept sucking, slowly at first, and then I heard him starting to swallow and gulp the milk down. I had to hold him in place for a bit while he took the milk off and once he tasted some breast milk, he just went for it. As the breast eased, I was able to take my hand away.

"Just keep him on for ten minutes and then we'll try the other side. I'll go and check on the others. I won't be long."

Mrs Lund had already given her baby the first side and had unwrapped her to try and wake her up for the second side.

"Are you able to take your baby back to the nursery for me when you've finished feeding?" I asked.

Mrs Lund was sitting up in bed and her baby was having a lovely feed. The baby had been breastfeeding well from the start and needed no test weighing or top ups. She had been ready to go home for a few days but, as she had other children at home, she was encouraged to stay in for the rest.

"Alright, I need to go to the loo anyway," she replied.

Mrs Aitken was managing her baby well and had got her baby on to the breast.

"Just three minutes each side and then give her the Karilac. It looks as if she knows what to do. What a little gem."

I went back to Mrs White and helped her to latch the baby to the other side. He had fed well. It was just her poor engorged breasts that were the problem. Once they settled down, she should be able to manage herself. I took the baby for a test weigh once he had finished feeding. Baby was 6lb 7oz when it went out and, after a feed, was 6lb 9oz. Two ounces – that's not bad.

"Your Mum has plenty of milk," I said to him as I changed him and tucked him in his cot.

Baby Lund was already in the nursery. I only had to get Baby Aitken in and they would all be fed and tucked down.

I grabbed the warmed breast pads and took them into Mrs White for her to put them on.

"Your baby got enough off you this time so there's no need to top him up. You have so much milk. Once your breasts have settled down, he should get on well and be away."

I was back in the office and all was quiet. I got my knitting out again. I must have knitted for an hour or so before I drifted off to sleep without realizing. Next thing, I was woken by the sound of the phone ringing. I startled, waking up from a deep sleep. I shook my head, wondering for a minute what the noise was and where I was.

"Hello, maternity annexe, Nurse speaking," I said hoping I wouldn't sound at all sleepy.

"It's Margaret Rowe here. I think my waters have broken. I got out of bed to go to the toilet and had this gush of fluid come out as I sat on the toilet. It kept going even after I finished. I have been having some pains since I went to bed, but I have been dozing in between as they weren't too bad."

"Can you put a pad on so we can see how much you are losing? You'll need to come in and be assessed," I was trying to think of what else to ask her when she just replied.

"Alright, we will have to organise the kids and then we'll come".

I quickly made a cup of tea and made my way over to the nurses' home to wake Sister. It took several loud knocks before she finally answered the door. A sleepy Sister Southgate opened the door dressed in a full-length, pink, flannelette nightie, with her long dark hair down past her shoulders. It was the only time I saw Sister Southgate with her hair down and not put up in a bun.

"Sister, Mrs Rowe is coming in. She says her waters have broken and she's been contracting since last night, although they didn't sound strong."

"Alright, I'll be over soon. Thanks." She took the cup of tea and shut the door.

I made my way back to maternity and started setting up the prep room and getting the labour room ready.

Mrs Rowe arrived soon after Sister. She appeared to be contracting quite strongly and needed to concentrate as each contraction came. Once Sister had shaved her and given the enema, I took the board off the bath and started running the water. The bath seemed to relax her as she sunk deep into the warm water.

"Oh, that's feels so good. Can I stay here for a while?"

"I think that will be alright. Just take your time." I left her, thinking how much the warm water seemed to help with the pain of the contractions. Mrs Rowe seemed relaxed as the water covered most of her body.

It was time for the early morning feed at 5am. I continued changing the babies and getting them out to their mums, while Sister looked after the labouring woman and did all the paperwork.

As soon as the babies were back in their cots, I started preparing the trolley for Mrs Aitken's perineal swab. I had become quicker at doing them now and it didn't take half an hour like it used to when I first started.

"This is the last swab you'll need," I said to her as I took the trolley into her room.

"Debbie will get you up this morning for a shower and, from then on, you'll be able to go down to the toilet yourself," I said to her as I finished.

By the time Debbie arrived for the morning shift, Mrs Rowe was in good labour and expected to give birth later in the morning.

As I walked out the door after getting changed, I thought the best part of night duty was getting into a nice warm bed while everyone else was going to work. I could climb into bed on a cold morning and just snuggle under the covers and sleep for most of the day.

A hot water bottle was my companion that I put my cold feet on in bed. I woke up in the middle of the afternoon and, even though I did have a good sleep, the feeling of being half asleep was with me until I had a shower, something to eat and a strong coffee.

I found out when I went to work for the next night shift that Margaret Rowe's baby was born as an undiagnosed breech. It was a footling breech, which is when the feet are presented first. This is a more difficult birth than a frank breech, which is when the bottom presents first.

A foot came out first and the baby's body was slowly pushed down by the contractions and the mother pushing. This became an emergency because, even though the body was delivered, the head got trapped behind the undilated cervix. It was a few minutes of trying to get the baby's head out and, when the baby was finally born, it was in a very poor condition and needed resuscitating.

Both Mrs Rowe and baby were rushed by ambulance to Palmerston North Hospital. Sister rang later that day to enquire about the baby. It was in the neonatal unit, still in a poor condition but stable. It was too early to tell whether the baby would have any lasting brain damage from the birth.

'What some women have to go through,' I thought. The woman didn't choose the outcome. It just seemed that some women had their babies with no problems at all, while others would have problems during the birth and the baby could be damaged as a result.

Life did not seem fair at times and, for some, their lives were full of nothing but lovely times, lovely births and healthy babies. For others, however, whose babies were damaged, their lives would be changed forever.

View from the Other Side

THREE MONTHS HAD PASSED SINCE the wedding. I was on duty one morning when I was overcome with nausea. I rushed to the toilet and threw up all my breakfast. I was a week overdue for my period and the nausea seemed to be confirmation that I was pregnant. We had both wanted to have a baby and were delighted with the prospect of becoming parents. Working in a maternity annexe, I was surrounded with babies and I had become quite clucky and wanted one of my own. It seemed a natural progression and many others our age were having children.

I went to Doctor Symes the next week and had to produce a urine sample. The sample had to be sent away for a frog test. A frog test involved injecting a sample of my urine into a female frog. If the frog produced eggs within 24 hours, it meant that I was pregnant. It was not until that evening that I was rung by Doctor Symes to say the test was positive and I was pregnant and to come and see him in the next month.

Both our parents were delighted when we broke the news to them and the mothers started knitting clothes at once for the expected baby. Rather than being daunted by the thought of becoming a mother, I couldn't wait.

I continued to work for as long as possible and finally finished work at 36 weeks. The next three weeks were spent washing nappies and preparing clothes and bedding for the new arrival. Being home without any pressure to go to work was lovely. It was enjoyable sleeping in and doing what I pleased. When I could, I spent a lot of time visiting Mum and my grandparents who lived just down the road. They loved my visits and, since Nana couldn't get out of the house, she appreciated me taking the time to see her and chat over a cup of tea. It had been five years since she had had both her legs amputated due to a secondary infection from diabetes. Anyone calling in was a break from the monotony of being inside unable to get out.

The weekly antenatal visits, when I would drive to the doctors' surgery for a checkup, came around every Tuesday morning. Apart from me putting on far too much weight, all had gone well.

When I went in for my check up at nearly 39 weeks, my blood pressure was up. It had steadily been creeping up since I had given up work. I was taken aback when Doctor Symes said that I needed to be admitted to hospital for bed rest until I had the baby. Even though I felt well, I was diagnosed with pre-eclampsia. I had all the classic signs of the disease, such as high blood pressure, oedema and protein in my urine.

I was in for bed rest for a week, which meant not being allowed to get out of bed except to have a bowel motion. The days dragged by, but I did have my knitting and would read the 'Women's Weekly' that Barry's mother had given me. She would get the magazine every week without fail. Mum came to see me every afternoon and Barry visited every evening. I had friends that would also visit in the afternoon. At the end of my first week in hospital, Doctor Symes decided to induce me three days before my due date.

I woke on the day of my induction with mild period-type pains. When I was panned and wiped, a large mucus plug was visible on the toilet paper. I was taken into the birthing suite to have my waters broken. I was given a shot of pethidine about twenty minutes before the procedure. When my legs were put up into the stirrups, I was so light headed and away with it, that having the hook put up inside me to puncture the bag of membranes was bearable. I felt the warm fluid pour out and a pad was put in place. I was wheeled back into my room to await events. It didn't take long before I was getting regular contractions that became stronger by the afternoon. They seemed to be starting in the front and coming around to the back. And as the contraction continued, the pain became stronger and stronger.

Once the contractions became very strong, I couldn't move and just lay on my side. I knew I should be more active and stand, so that at least gravity was on my side. But it was enough to cope with the pain itself. I would shut my eyes and lie still with each contraction, almost paralysed by the pain. I just lay there on my side and breathed the best I could until the contraction past.

Our son was born at 9:21pm that same day on the 6th of July 1972. I sustained an episiotomy – an incision made into the perineum to make the opening bigger, allowing the baby's head to come through more easily – like most women who had a baby in the 1970s did. The worst thing was hearing the scissors opening and shutting, while Doctor Symes waited for the next contraction.

"I know what you are going to do with those," I said, raising my head and looking at the person holding the scissors.

There was a roar of laughter, with all in the room finding it extremely funny. The inevitable came as I lay down again. I felt the overwhelming urge to push as the contraction came and heard the sound of crunching as the scissors cut through my flesh. Surprisingly, the pain was no worse than what I had already been feeling. I just wanted to get this baby out. So with an almighty push, the head was born. And then another push and my baby boy arrived.

As he was wheeled back to the labour room beside me, I lay back and looked down at him. He had big, wide, blues eyes and seemed to be looking around as if he had been here before and was taking it all in. Barry looked at him and smiled. We continued to just gaze upon this new little person as we drank our tea and ate the toast that was brought to us. I leaned down, picked him up and started undressing him, examining every part of the baby we had created.

"Look at his feet. They are Wilson feet. See how long they are," Barry said, referring to his ancestor on his father's side.

I was relieved, excited and overwhelmed.

"He's so beautiful, isn't he?" I said to Barry as we gazed down at him lying in his crib.

I picked him up and started to dress our little baby boy as he squirmed, trying to put his fists in his mouth. I put a little singlet and gown on him, feeling his long, blonde hair as I put the clothing over his head. Hair that was so fair it could hardly be seen. Yet when you felt it, there was a crop of hair to the nape of his neck.

Sister McLaren came in as I finished putting the nappy on.

"Do you want to try and feed him? You are going to try and breastfeed him, aren't you? He looks as if he would go on and he is so alert at the moment," she said.

I started to lift up the hospital gown I had on and instinctively positioned him to go on my left breast.

I was pleasantly surprised that with little effort he opened his mouth and as I brought him onto my breast, he started to suck. Slowly at first, then gathering momentum as the sucking got stronger and more rhythmical. I sat up, not moving in case I disturbed this perfect moment. He knew what to do and I wanted to savour the moment forever as the feeding continued unabated.

We were off to a good start and after sucking steadily for a few minutes he slowed down and came off. We were wheeled down to the postnatal room I was to be in. It was the last room on the left by the door. There was another girl in the room who had birthed a baby girl earlier in the day. I knew her from when I went to primary school.

Barry left and finally I went to sleep. My newborn was taken to the nursery with all the other babies, lined up along the wall. Betty came in and woke me up for a swab at 4am. How nice it was to be freshened up. It was so soothing to have warm Savlon poured down the area that had taken such a beating. As she bound me up again, I asked for some paracetamol. The local anaesthetic had well and truly worn off and from the waist down it felt like I'd been run over by a bus.

"I will let your baby sleep, Julie, and will give him some Karilac next feed, so you can go back to sleep till breakfast time. You won't have to worry about feeding him till the nine o'clock feed."

Part of me was pleased to just curl up again and I didn't argue. I still felt exhausted and was happy to get as much sleep as I could.

Christine brought my son to me the next morning for the nine o'clock feed. I was not allowed out of bed for 24 hours, so had to wait for the baby to be brought to me. Christine beamed from ear to ear as she handed him to me.

"You were clever weren't you to have a baby boy. See if you can get him on yourself. I'll be back after I get the other babies out."

With that, she left me to it.

"Well I should know what to do," I thought. "After all, I have been working here for over two years now."

I tried to wake the little one up but he was not having a bar of it and as much as I undressed him, blew on him and played with his ears he would not wake up. He was not interested in feeding at all. He was out to it and didn't even flinch. I had given up by the time Christine came back.

"How did you get on? Did he go on ok?" she asked

"He hasn't gone on at all," I replied. "I have tried everything to wake him up, but he's just not interested."

"Keep trying. I'll go and get the Karilac for him and you can give him that. Maybe he'll wake up next feed."

I still had no success waking him up before Christine arrived back with the Karilac.

"Just give him this," she said. "I'll be back soon to collect the bottle and the baby."

I took the bottle and worked the teat into his mouth. He took the bottle without any problem or fuss. Within a few minutes, the contents of the bottle were gone.

The same scenario was repeated every four hours. At each feed, he was uninterested in going on the breast, but would eagerly take the bottle. I continued to try and be positive. After all, it was only the first day and it is normal for the baby to be sleepy.

Barry visited after work.

"What do you think we should call him?" He said.

The second name, Haigh, was non-negotiable, as it had been in Barry's family for five generations. Definitely the second name would be Haigh. That had been already decided. Barry had a childhood friend called Kelvin and Barry and I both liked the name, so we decided on the name Kelvin Haigh Watson. Nicer than calling the baby 'it' or 'him'. We were both still on cloud nine and Barry had a grin from ear to ear.

"Your Dad was wondering about wetting the baby's head this Friday night at the RSA, so I won't come and see you that night. Are you alright with that?" He asked.

"Yes, that's ok. Mum came up today and Dad is coming to see me tomorrow. He is so chuffed with having his first grandchild and it being a boy. He is already talking about taking him fishing and teaching him to play golf."

I enjoyed Barry's visits and having that time with him. I looked forward to him coming every day to see me and filling me in with what was happening. He was not too bad at cooking a meal. Very basic, but he wouldn't starve. Mum and his mother, though, were making sure he didn't and each night he seemed to have somewhere to go for his evening meal.

He was a man of the age, as his mother had always done everything for him. She was still making his bed for him when I met him and, up until we were married, he had never had to wash his clothes. He never had to do many domestic duties apart from wash or dry the dishes. A chore he shared with his sister when she lived at home.

Barry did his fair share of work on the farm though, and had plenty of jobs to do. He was still mowing his grandmother's lawn every week, so I could forgive the domestic side of things.

The following morning I was pleased to be able to get out of bed. I was escorted down to the shower and toilet as if I had had a major operation and needed to take it slowly and be shown what to do and how to do it. I did already know the procedure, but as I was now a patient, I had to be shown regardless of what I knew. Even if you were having your eighth baby, it would still be the same.

As I got out of bed, it felt like my stomach and excess flab had just fallen on the floor. I felt a bit weak and shaky as I was led down the corridor. I was taken into the toilet where I was undressed from the waist down. All the paraphernalia came off – the abdominal binder with all the pins, the material pad and the normal pad.

"I know you have worked here, but I still have to show you this," said Leanne, who had started since I had left about four weeks ago.

I felt rather insulted that she deemed it necessary to go into so much detail.

'I suppose she is new and wants to do it right,' I thought to myself. 'At least now I will be free to walk around and do what I please instead of being confined to bed.'

I had been in bed far too long, as I hadn't been allowed up since being admitted over a week ago.

The routine of the annexe was pretty tight and regimented but at least I could walk around, go into the dining room for meals and go and use the phone, which was by the labour room.

Baby feeding times were every four hours at 9am, 1pm, 5pm, 9pm, 1am and 5am. Breakfast was at 7:30am, the main meal of the day was at midday and tea was at 5:30pm. Morning tea was at 10am and afternoon tea was at 3pm. Nap time was from 10:30-11:30am, when we had a compulsory lie down on our tummies. The physiotherapist came and took exercises in the dining room at 11:30am before lunch. Visiting times were 2-4pm for the general public and husbands could visit from 7-8pm. No one else was allowed in without special permission. So there wasn't a lot of free time at all really. It seemed every minute was accounted for and I had to fit in going to the toilet and having a shower in between.

It was the day three and Kelvin still had not been back on the breast. I was starting to get worried about it and every time he refused to go on the breast he was given a supplement. I was getting some help now from the sisters, but no one was having success and my anxiety was building every time he went back to the nursery after another failed attempt. The third day was test weigh time and with each test weigh, there was a minimal result. At best, about half a teaspoon was the result of a few sucking attempts.

Sister Foster was on the next day and decided she was going to sort out the problem.

"Right," she said. "We won't give him any extra today and get him really hungry. Maybe starving him will do it."

With that, she left the room. What a morning! With each feed he still wouldn't go on the breast. And as Sister Foster had set herself a challenge, Kelvin was taken back to the nursery without a feed. After the 1pm feed and before the visitors arrived, I went to the toilet. Looking over to the nursery, I could see his blankets moving and as I went over to the nursery window, I could see his face red and screaming.

Sister Foster was in the office reading the paper.

"He's crying really hard," I said as I walked into the office to talk to her about my concerns.

"He'll be fine. By next feed he'll be hungry enough to go on, so we'll wait till then. It's no good trying him now."

I felt powerless and unable to do what all my motherly instincts were telling me to do. I made my way back to my room feeling worried and anxious, unable to help my baby who I felt was crying out for his mother.

My visitors took my mind off the problem for a time, but when the 5pm feed came around, I almost dreaded the disappointment again.

Sister McLaren was on for the afternoon shift. Sister Foster had told her the plan of letting him starve until he got so hungry that he would be so eager to breastfeed and he would go on with no problem.

The problem was, however, that being in the nursery for four hours without having a feed made him more frustrated, since the cues for feeding were being ignored.

By the time feed time came around, Kelvin was exhausted from crying himself to sleep and, no matter how hard I tried, I could not wake him. The time when he would have gone on the breast when he was hungry and not frustrated had long past. With each feed, he became sleepier and tired from crying and not having his needs met.

Sister McLaren brought him to me and, as she started to try and wake him for a feed and get him interested in feeding off the breast, I burst into tears.

"I want to put him on the bottle. He's starving," I cried.

"Are you sure, Julie? He is alright and I might be able to get him on you."

"No," I said "I've made up my mind. I can't continue like this. I want him to have a feed and I have decided I'm going to put him on the bottle."

By this time, I was so anxious and worried. I just wanted him to have a feed any way he could.

"Well, if you're sure. It's your decision and we are happy if you want to bottle feed him." Poor Sister McLaren was trying her best and it was unfortunate that she had come on duty when the damage had been done.

I really wanted to breastfeed my baby, but to have him down in the nursery, knowing that he was crying and unsettled, until the next feed time was more than I could cope with.

Certainly my experience was not an isolated one. Many mothers, overcome with anxiety at their baby's crying and distress in a maternity nursery, threw in the towel and resorted to feeding their baby formula from a bottle.

It wasn't until the 1980s that rooming in was brought in, so that the baby was by their mother's bed all the time, even during the night, allowing mother and baby to have undisturbed access to each other.

Even though the four hourly routine still continued for a time, the babies that became unsettled could still have another breastfeed or at least be held by their mothers. Slowly things started to change and baby-led feeding became the norm. Test weighing stopped and assessment of whether a baby was getting enough breast milk was based on how settled the baby was, how often the baby passed urine and the colour and the frequency of their bowel movements. The mother was listened to as women's maternal instinct rose to the fore.

Renovations

L<small>IFE COULD NOT HAVE BEEN</small> more perfect when we brought our new baby home. We were so proud and thrilled to have this little boy in our lives. I couldn't imagine life being any better. Barry and I were so happy to be parents and excited about looking after and caring for him. We wanted the best for him and to give our new baby the best start in life. Our parents were supportive as well. They were generous with knitting clothes for him and were frequent visitors to see how we were.

When we arrived home from the maternity home, we laid our little baby in the cane bassinet that had been bought especially for him. We had bought it second hand from a woman in Palmerston North and were pleased that we had found a cane bassinet in such good condition. Barry spray painted the bassinet white to freshen it up. I made a fine, white net skirt, which was gathered at the top and flowed down to the ground. The inside I lined with white satin and the mattress sat snugly inside. Both the bassinet and the baby it held stayed by our bed for the first few months, until Kelvin grew out of it and we put him in a cot in his own room.

Barry's mother made sheets for both the bassinet and the cot from old sheets that she had. She made them to the right size, some for summer and flannelette ones for the winter. Soon after we were home, Barry's parents came around one night to see us. Barry's mother handed me a parcel as they sat down in the lounge. I undid the wrapping and opened the paper to find a covering of white tissue paper. As I took off the tissue paper, a hand knitted, white, woollen shawl was revealed.

"How beautiful," I said as I opened the soft woollen shawl to see the full extent of the work that had been created.

"This must have taken hours to knit." I gazed at the intricate detail, which was so fine and exquisite.

"She started it as soon as she knew the baby was coming," said Barry's father.

For every grandchild, Barry's mother knitted a woollen shawl as something that could be handed down to the generations to come.

From the first night home, I had to get used to getting up in the middle of the night to feed a hungry, crying baby. Kelvin woke two or three times a night and would not stop crying until he was satisfied with a bottle of milk. My deep sleep would be disturbed by the crying baby, who was oblivious to the freezing cold outside. His mother would have to get up, boil a jug of water to heat the bottle and then climb back into bed to feed him. Once drunk, though, he would be satisfied for another three or four hours. Barry seemed to sleep through any disturbance. The crying baby in the dead of the night, the bed lamp going on, me getting out of bed to get the bottle, returning, getting into bed again, and then feeding our little baby would never disturb him. I didn't try and be quiet, yet as the bed light lit up the room and the baby cried until the milk satisfied him, Barry slept on.

I was a bit peeved that nothing seemed to disturb or wake him, but then subconsciously maybe he knew that I was tending to his son – it was 'women's work', after all.

'Fortunately your mother is here or you would never be heard or get fed,' I thought as I climbed into bed with my little baby.

The house was freezing, especially at night when I got up for the night feeds. It was built in the 1930s and had never had anything done to it, so it was in dire need of a makeover. It was very cold with unsatisfactory heating. The house had high ceilings and there was no insulation. The fire place in the lounge was small and even though there were fireplaces in every bedroom it was not practical to go around lighting fires in every room. The night store heater we put in had improved things but not nearly enough. It was still very cold. The walls were lined with scrim, which made the house very drafty and the wallpaper was very outdated. We decided that the house needed renovating to make it warmer and more comfortable.

Barry had some lessons from his mother on how to wallpaper and soon became an expert at matching wallpaper as he applied it. Most of the wallpaper we chose had large medallion patterns and each room had a different colour and theme.

The lounge we did in cream with large, gold medallion wallpaper. I made full-length, gold, crushed velvet curtains that fell at either side of the large bay window at the end of the room. The bay window was made of four smaller windows that all had stained glass fan lights above. The room looked so grand once we had finished it. A door, which led to the veranda, also had a stained glass window at the top.

The stained glass windows were set off by the newly decorated room and looked so beautiful and ornate. The room had a high

127

ceiling with varnished beams in sections. In between the beams there was smooth plaster that we painted white, which accentuated the dark, varnished beams. We replaced the open fire in the lounge with a wood burner for the cold winters and the fireplaces in all the bedrooms were taken out.

Before winter, Barry and his father spent a few weekends gathering and cutting firewood from the farm. They did enough for both houses and we had firewood stacked high in the wood shed.

We decided to put wallpaper above the wood panelling that went around the middle of the hallway. From the wood panelling to the skirting board at the bottom, we put plainer wallpaper that matched the wallpaper at the top. It looked so lovely when it was finished and showed off the beautiful woodwork in the hall.

In the bathroom, we got rid of the old bath that had legs and put in a modern one with a new vanity, toilet and lino. In time, we also put in large sliding doors off the kitchen, which led to a concrete patio and, off that, we built a new laundry. Old wooden buildings outside had a copper and concrete tubs for doing the laundry, so they needed to go. Dad was happy to take the copper out to the bach for boiling up the crayfish. The 1930s look was soon replaced with a modern 1970s look.

Over the next few months, we spent all our spare money and time decorating the house and putting our stamp on it. With each room, we would paint the ceilings, put new wallpaper up, put up new curtains and, eventually, lay new carpet. A few months after Kelvin was born, I went back to work at the maternity annexe, doing about two shifts a week to help fund all the renovations we were doing and buy other things we needed for the house.

Barry's mother and my mother were only too willing to help care for Kelvin when I went back to work. When I worked in the weekends, Barry would mind Kelvin. So it worked out well and was not too much effort juggling both home and work.

Nothing much had changed in maternity and the same staff was still there, so it was easy going back to the familiar. I was fortunate that I was able to just slip back into work with no problem. I didn't even have to have an interview. I just rang to say when I could work and I was back.

The work continued and we began thinking of having another baby. We wanted four and were off to a good start. We didn't want to waste any time and when Kelvin was eight months old, I was pregnant again.

Born for Life

Shelley

I WAS FEELING TIRED AND heavy, with only three weeks to go before I was due to have baby number two. We had been trying to pick carpet for the house and I was so worried about making the wrong decision. The carpet had been chosen and it was going to be laid in the next few days. But even after Barry and I made the decision, I was worrying about whether we had made the right choice. The carpet was so expensive. I absolutely loved our house and we had worked all that year doing up every room. The carpet was going to be the finishing touch.

I went up town for a walk the day before my next doctor's appointment, which was now each week. As I sat down on one of the park benches in the square up town, I felt breathless and not well. Kelvin was sixteen months old and a little live wire. It took all my energy to make sure he stayed in his push chair. He wanted to get out and run around up Main Street. I was finding it harder to look after him in my heavily pregnant state.

The following day was my antenatal appointment and, after taking my blood pressure and testing my urine, Doctor Symes said, "Go home and pack your bags, as you need to be admitted to hospital for bed rest."

I was not that surprised to have pre-eclampsia again after having it with Kelvin and felt quite relieved that there was a reason I had been feeling nauseous and unwell. Back home, I waited for Barry to finish work so he could take me up to the hospital.

We came to the door of the annexe and were greeted by Sister Foster.

"Come with me," she said and led me into the second antenatal room.

I got dressed into one of my nighties and got into the clean, cold, white sheets. Barry stayed for about an hour before he had to go home to see to Kelvin, whom he had dropped off at his mother's place.

He had to make arrangements for Kelvin to be looked after while I was in hospital. It was a juggling act between my parents and Barry's parents while Barry went to work. Then he would look after Kelvin after he finished work.

I was on bed rest and only allowed up to go to the toilet to have a bowel motion and, even then, I had to go out in a wheelchair. It was complete bed rest, even down to the bed sponges. I was put on medication the next morning as my blood pressure was showing no signs of coming down.

For three weeks, I lay in bed looking out at the rose gardens and the beautifully manicured lawn. Every morning, Doctor Symes would come in at eight o'clock to see me. Each day, I would wait in anticipation for some good news, like him saying I could get out of bed and have a walk around the gardens, but that was not to be.

I looked forward to anything that took the monotony away. Morning and afternoon tea, the meals, and chats with Smithy as she gave the trays out and then came and got them. Every day at two o'clock visiting time, Mum very faithfully brought Kelvin up to see me. Barry used to come when he could, usually after work before going home to get his tea.

The sisters used to come in regularly to take my blood pressure and listen to the baby's heartbeat. Sometimes they would sit down and stop for a chat, which was nice. Three weeks was a long time to be confined to bed, so I became excited when Doctor Symes came in one morning to say that I would be induced the next day. He looked concerned as he told me that my blood test had come back. The results meant the placenta had stopped working efficiently and the baby needed to be born.

At last, my time of being confined to bed was coming to an end. I could hardly sleep with the anticipation of a new baby and an end to being stuck in bed. The next day, I was wheeled into the birthing room and put up in stirrups for the procedure of rupturing my membranes. As it was a difficult procedure, I was given pethidine to relax me and to help accomplish the task.

Being strung up in the stirrups with all my lower body exposed was not that easy, but the prospect of the outcome outweighed any embarrassment I would have normally felt. I had my legs splayed out for all to see, but I felt indifferent as the pethidine took effect. I felt pushing and poking as Doctor Symes put his fingers up my vagina to find my cervix. Not an easy thing, but with a final push of the amnihook, the fluid flowed out.

"There. All done," he said in a satisfied tone. "Well, that should do it and you should go into labour today."

He then left it to Sister Drury and Christine to take me back to my room for the long wait.

"Try and sit up in bed as much as you can today and let the water just keep draining out," Sister said as I was wheeled back to my room.

Despite all my enthusiasm and with all the will in the world, nothing happened all day. I was still on top of the world knowing that, even though nothing was happening, the baby could not stay there forever. It had its marching orders. I couldn't help but feel that the baby also wanted out, as I felt some very violent kicking that day. I was concerned at the time but didn't say anything as it settled down again later that day.

Mum came up to see me in the afternoon and was surprised when she saw I was still in the same room.

"I thought you'd be in the labour room by now," she said.

No, nothing's happening yet. Not even a twinge, so it might not be today unless I do something tonight."

"Nana and Grandad are asking how you are and are at home waiting for some news."

The anticipation was building and expectations were high, but nothing happened all that day. I finally fell asleep that night and, surprisingly, woke in the morning still in one piece and with no contractions.

I wasn't allowed breakfast and was wheeled into the labour room to wait for the doctor to arrive. Doctor Symes came in at the normal time and the plan was set. I was to have a drip put in my vein with syntocinon put through to get the contractions going. Sister Drury was on again and helped put the cannula in my left hand. Then I was attached to the bag containing the drug that was going to force this baby to come out. Syntocinon is a drug that causes the uterus to contract in the same way that oxytocin naturally occurs and causes contractions when a woman goes into labour.

Every fifteen minutes or so, Sister Drury would come in to count the drops of syntocinon that were going into my vein, and would listen to the baby's heartbeat with the pinard. I could not hear the heartbeat myself, but every time there was either no comment or a "that's fine."

Doctor Symes came in at lunch time to check on progress and I was having a few tightenings by then. He also listened to the heartbeat. All seemed to be on track for the birth of my second baby. Sister McLaren was on for the afternoon shift and on her way to the office she poked her head in to see how it was all going.

The contractions had started to get stronger and now I was lying on my side, hardly able to move with the contractions. I was trying to cope with the pain, thinking of all the people out there somewhere who weren't in any pain at all and wishing I was one of them. The drip was still going and it had worked – the contractions were intense now. The drip wasn't being increased anymore but was kept at the same level so the contractions would keep coming. They were coming like waves in the sea and there was no stopping them now or the intensity of them. Sister McLaren was coming in often now and listening to the heartbeat.

How I hated it when she would say, "Roll on your back so I can hear the baby." Then she would press so hard into my lower abdomen, as if she was pushing the baby to the other side and through my back.

I was trying to remember to breathe, "Huh, huh whew." I was trying to remember what I used to say to women when I had looked after them in labour.

I was trying to talk to myself. 'Just go with it. It's like climbing a mountain. You reach the top and then you come down the other side,' I kept saying to myself. Barry was there now and holding my hand.

Every time a contraction started, I took hold of his hand and squeezed as hard as I could, closing my eyes to cope with the pain. I would open them to see a man who was full of fear and worry. It was hard to cope with someone he loved being in so much pain.

"I can't do any more, I can't do any more," I cried. "Can't you stop the drip, I can't take it. Please I can't take it."

Lying on my side, I just kept my eyes closed and squeezed and squeezed. I started to grunt and "Mmmuuh, mmmuuuh."

"Quick! Move her into theatre," I heard Sister say to Christine as they battled with the doors and the drip, trying to get everything through the doors. Barry helped them hold the doors open and guide the bed. Once the bed and drip made it through, Barry retreated behind the closed doors.

"Ring Doctor Symes," I heard Sister say to Christine as she had said to me many times before.

I just laid there and with every wave of the contraction, I felt the urge to move my bowels. I didn't think about anything but just doing what my body was ordering me to do. I had no control but just tried to go with my body.

"Huhu, huhu. I need some water," I called out to anyone that would listen.

Christine came over and placed the glass of water to my lips. Half of it went down by neck but it was cold.

"How is she going, Sister? How long has she been in second

stage?" I heard Doctor Symes say as the familiar banging of the theatre doors went back and forth.

"She's not been pushing long but since it's her second baby, I thought I would call you now," Sister McLaren replied.

"It looks as if it won't be too long. We'll see with the next contraction," and with that I heard the clearing of his throat. "Has the heartbeat been alright, Sister?"

"Yes, it has been alright," was the reply. With that, the next wave came and I pushed with everything I had.

'Here it comes, here it comes,' I thought and, with that, the head was born and next was the final push.

Finally, the relief. 'The baby is here,' I thought.

For a brief moment the excitement was back, but then the baby was gone and there was no sound, just a sense of panic came into the room. I looked to see the baby being hastily taken to the resuscitaire and the frantic rush of everyone there. I could hear no sound but a list of instructions being given out by the Doctor.

'Don't cry out, don't cry out,' I kept saying to myself. 'Don't distract them, don't distract them,' I kept saying to myself, fighting back the tears as I watched in disbelief, not really believing what I was seeing.

I looked over to see a baby, fully developed and fully grown with long, dark, black hair. I could see she was a little girl struggling to live, but not winning, not making it into this world. I saw a baby, who was born silent and unable to move or make a sound. I could see Doctor and Sister trying to get her to respond, but the baby was not responding. I lay in silence as I saw my precious baby girl not make it into this world. I was lying numb, not knowing what was happening, not knowing what to say or do. Christine came over to me and held my hand and then the doctor instructed that I be taken out of the room.

I lay there alone in the labour room as they went back into theatre to continue working on the baby. I could not believe what was happening. I was stunned and just lay in silence. Barry was nowhere. I found out later that he was waiting in the corridor and only knew about our baby dying as I was wheeled down the corridor to the postnatal room.

"She died. She didn't live," I called to him as I was wheeled down with Barry following behind. He had waited for hours in the corridor not knowing what was happening. No one had gone to get him. They must have forgotten he was there.

After a time, Sister McLaren came into the labour room where I was. My baby had not made it. She had not cried or come into this world. She was dead.

"I'm sorry," she said.

"Can I hold her?" I said as I tried to force back the tears.

"Oh, no don't," she said, as if holding my baby would be a thing that I might regret in the future. Like it was better not to hold her, like I would not be able to handle it and it would not be good for me to do so.

I didn't argue. I thought Sister McLaren must know the best thing for me to do and that it was best not to hold my daughter whom I had longed for all these months. The baby, for whom I had waited so long and lay in a hospital bed for the past three weeks.

I had longed for a girl. I had longed for a daughter. To see her grow up, to go shopping with her, to take her to ballet, to let her play the piano and ride horses. I was going to let my daughter do all the things I was never able to do.

She was going to have the best of everything we could give her – nice clothes, a good education. My daughter was going to be whatever she wanted to be. I was going to encourage her to be the best she could at whatever she wanted to be. I burst into tears, as it was all over for her before it even began. A new life had gone before any dreams could happen or even begin.

Doctor Symes came in looking very ashen and drawn. He pulled up a chair by my bed.

"I don't know what I would do if Angela and I had lost a baby," he said, pondering what it would be like for him and his wife if the same tragedy had happened to them.

"Her heart beat for 25 minutes but she just didn't respond. I could have kept going but you are a mother for 60 years. It is a long time and she would have been very brain damaged."

I just listened, still stunned with what was happening.

"Why did it happen?" I said.

"There was a knot in the cord," he said. "I think that with everything else it was just the straw that broke the camel's back. With your high blood pressure and the pre-eclampsia, it was the last straw.

"The knot was loose though. It was very loose," Sister McLaren chipped in.

"I thought only obese people got high blood pressure," I said. "How is it that I have it?"

"Well, all size people get high blood pressure. Big, small, thin, fat," he said with the strain showing on his face.

I didn't say much, just tried to make sense of it all and wondered how this could happen. I started to sob relentlessly. I was put down in one of the double rooms on my own. In the morning, word had got around about what had happened. All the staff that I knew and had worked with came in to offer their sympathy and support.

Sister Foster, who was on in the morning, came down to my room and said how sorry she was. They all went over to the morgue and came back and described her to me. One by one, the reports came back.

"She is so beautiful, Julie. She looks so much like you. She has dark hair. Beautiful, long, dark hair," they said.

The reports kept coming all day as, one by one, they went over to see her and then reported back to me how beautiful she looked. I never asked again about going to see her. The word, I felt, had been final. I had no say in the matter. Barry went the next day to register the birth and the death. We had decided on a name before she was born. It was to be Shelley Anne Watson and so we named her.

Barry went to see the undertaker about the funeral. A big debate started between the undertaker and Doctor Symes as to whether she had lived or was a stillborn. The undertaker thought she was stillborn and should be buried in an unmarked grave along the fence line at the cemetery with no gravestone or recognition.

Doctor Symes argued that her heart had beaten for 25 minutes after birth and that she had a slight reflex when she was born, so she should have a proper burial and gravestone. We wanted her to be buried properly and have a gravestone so we could visit her grave and acknowledge that she did exist, even though she had not lived.

Doctor Symes won the argument and she was to be buried on the fifth day. Barry dealt with all that side of things and came in as much as he could to visit me. I had a double room to myself even though I was in the postnatal area. One night it got too much and I just cried all night, despairing at my loss, wondering how people can have children and neglect them. Here we were with our hearts open to have a baby and she had died. It made no sense to me. It was totally unfair.

The day before the funeral I asked about going out on leave so I could be there. By this time, I had been in hospital for four days and there was no sign of me being released. The answer was "no" from Doctor Symes.

Sister McLaren asked him for me and came back to tell me I was not allowed to attend the funeral. The decision was made with no reason given, just a big fat "no". The final word was spoken and no one questioned or argued my case to go.

I look back and wonder why I just took that and did not say anything. I was only twenty years old and had always been brought up to obey those in authority and never question the decisions they made.

Doctors were revered and they supposedly knew what was best for their patients and made decisions for them. The doctors had the last and final word on everything. Nothing was questioned. The doctor knew best and his decision was final.

I looked out the window on the day of the funeral and wondered how it was going. Smithy brought me in a cup of tea and stood with me for a bit while I gazed out the window, tears rolling down my face.

"Why could I not be there? I am her mother," I said.

Life continued in the postnatal ward. Women came in, had their babies, stayed for a few days and then went home. I was still in. I don't know why and I was never told. The word hadn't been given for me to go home yet. I was an inpatient and had no baby to care for. I was just doing the hospital stay, surrounded by vases of flowers and cards that flooded the room. They were on every shelf and trolley in the room. Every night, all the flowers were taken out of my room and lined up along the corridor.

Finally, I was released from hospital a week after Shelley was born. She had been born on the Saturday night and I was discharged the following Saturday. Barry came to get me with Kelvin. As I walked in the door of our home, all I could feel was loss and all the dreams of bringing home a new baby that were now shattered.

Dark Days

WALKING INTO THE HOUSE BROUGHT it home again. The signs of an expected new arrival were all still present – the empty bassinet waiting for the new baby, all the new baby clothes on the bed. Cards and flowers had arrived during the week and were on the kitchen bench as I walked in.

Kelvin jumped around, excited his mum was home. I had been away four weeks and his excitement was plain to see. He had no idea what had gone on and was too young to try and explain it to. Mum had potty trained him in my absence and, even at night, he didn't need a nappy anymore.

During the first month of being home, I got a few messages from others who had experienced the same trauma. They were mainly friends of Mum and Dad who had also lost babies during childbirth. It was more common when Mum was having children. A few women Mum knew contacted me to express their sympathy and just to say I was not alone and that the same tragedy had happened to them.

I rang my grandmother while in hospital and she said, "Yes, I had a baby die as well. I know how you are feeling."

She was so loving and caring. She never saw her baby either. She didn't even know what the sex of her baby was, but she always felt sure it was the baby boy she never had. She had two girls and her third baby had died. I used to go and visit Nana and Grandad regularly. They lived just a few houses away and I loved going to see them and having a cup of tea. They were close to me all my life, as we used to stay there a lot when we were children.

Shelley had died on the 15th of December 1973 and I was out of hospital a few days before Christmas day. I had bought all the Christmas presents, including a present for the new baby, before going into hospital. I knew I would be busy with a baby right on Christmas, so I was all organised for it. All the presents were there as a reminder of the wonderful Christmas that we had expected with the new baby.

That night, Dad suggested that we go out for dinner at the RSA for his birthday, which was on the 21st of December. We all went for dinner while Kelvin was looked after by Barry's parents. There was an atmosphere of quiet grief that night.

We sat down and ordered our dinner. Dad got up and went to order some drinks. The atmosphere was tense and no one seemed happy or to be enjoying themselves.

Barry said something and I snapped at him. Dad sprung to his defence as he returned and put the drinks on the table.

"Leave Barry alone," he said. "He has been so busy while you've been in hospital. He's not had a minute to himself."

My heart sank. I hadn't meant anything by it. I was just so stressed. I know it had been hard on him as well. He had to organise the funeral and all the arrangements after Shelley died. He also had to keep working, as he had no one to take over from him. We did a rural mail run and had to deliver mail to the farmers regardless of what was happening in our lives. It was a contract we had to keep.

I felt hurt, though, that Dad had taken Barry's side. I was so stunned that he hadn't understood how I was feeling. I didn't say anything, but just grieved inside about how he had spoken to me. It was so unlike Dad, as he never told us off or even commented on matters. Normally he was so placid and relaxed. There was tension in the air, with everyone coping in their own way with what had happened.

There was no crying or displays of emotion, just tension. I was quiet during the dinner, not wanting to say anything. I was crying inside about the lack of support and comfort I was getting.

No one talked about Shelley or what had happened. That was how it was going to be from then on. There were no comments, no acknowledgement of her existence. Life went back to normal and I was expected to just get on with it and forget it ever happened.

The notes, letters and cards came for about two weeks but it was soon quiet. Marcia, my friend and bridesmaid, had left to live in Australia a few months before and others that I had known had moved away from Pahiatua. I had the occasional visit from friends but very soon I felt very alone. Barry and the rest of the family didn't want to talk about it. It was as if Shelley had never been born. Barry continued to do the rural mail run and I went back to looking after Kelvin full time, keeping the house, doing the meals, gardening and shopping.

For a time, I coped well. But it didn't last. After everything settled down and supposedly life was back to normal, the depression started. No one saw me when I was alone in my room, crying for hours at a time and not coping at all. I had no one to talk to about how I was feeling, no one to help me. I felt that no one cared.

I thought I had loads of friends before I had Shelley, but after a few months, I felt I had no one. People stayed away, as it was too hard to come and see me after what had happened. No one knew how I was struggling, as I kept it to myself. When people did see me, they thought I was fine.

I spent hours on my own at home. Barry would come home late. Sometimes he would come in and, when he saw I was upset, he would go out again and not return for hours. When he hadn't come home and it was getting dark, I would go to the corner of the street, crying my eyes out, to see if I could see him coming.

He couldn't cope with my tears, so he would just go out. The feelings of loneliness and lack of support and care left me wanting to kill myself.

I would sit in my room when Kelvin was having his sleeps, planning and imagining how I was going to do it. Slitting my wrists, I thought, would be easiest, but then there would be the mess of all the blood. I would have to do it outside on the grass because I didn't want to ruin the new carpet. I just didn't want to be in this pain anymore. I didn't want to be in this world. My thoughts of self-destruction would always be stopped with thoughts of Kelvin. They would always bring me back to my senses.

I could not leave him without a mother. He was only eighteen months old so I had to just keep going and endure the pain. My thoughts went from despair and suicide to obsessing about having another baby. I desperately wanted to get pregnant again, but it wasn't happening.

My relationship with Barry was distant but I needed him to have another baby. I had lost interest in everything else in life and the goal that controlled me was having another baby.

I went back to Doctor Symes for help and started crying in his room, I was so desperate, filled with grief and loss. I wanted another baby but it wasn't happening. I burst into tears, so he wrote out a script for some medication.

I got the script filled and took the medication when I got home. It was late morning and it didn't take long to work. Before long, I didn't care about anything and didn't really know what was going on.

I went into the lounge, sat in the chair there and closed my eyes. I felt lightheaded and drowsy with not a care in the world. I then spent the next hour or two spaced out for the afternoon on the couch. Kelvin was running around outside and I didn't know where he was or have the energy to care. After a time, I shook my head, got up out of the chair and went looking for him. He was running around outside in the front of the house with the gate open. I grabbed him and carried him inside.

I reached up to the cupboard and got the tablets that were meant to help me and tipped them in the rubbish, knowing that I couldn't take them again. One tablet had rendered me hopeless and unable to function properly. I knew it was not the answer and I just had to tough it out somehow.

Day after day, I had to fight my emotions. Each day when I put Kelvin down for his sleep in the afternoon, I would go to my room and cry for my lost baby. I was so low and depressed and no one seemed to notice.

I wanted to leave Barry, but had nowhere to go and no one to turn to. And how could I leave? I felt I couldn't hurt Mum and Dad, who had spent all that money putting on a lovely wedding. They had let me get married, despite all the criticism they got for letting me get married at seventeen years old.

Shelley had died in December and, in the following September, my period was late. Dare I hope that I was pregnant again? It was about a week late and I was getting my hopes up that perhaps another baby was on the way. I made an appointment to see Doctor Symes on the Monday morning. I knew it was early, but maybe he could confirm it for me and give me some hope that would help me feel like living again. It was the Saturday morning before the appointment and on Saturday I always did most of the housework. I did the vacuuming, washed the floors, cleaned the bathroom and changed all the sheets. I was very energetic that morning and probably did more than normal. Perhaps it was the thought of being pregnant that gave me renewed energy.

I took all the sheets off the bed, went to put the washing in the washing machine and was in the bedroom putting the new sheets on when the first pains came. I called out for Barry to help me, went and sat in the lounge and tried to rest and calm down.

The waves of pain kept coming. I just tried to keep calm and not move. Why did I work so hard? Why did I do all that work this morning? I didn't have to. Barry made me a cup of tea and I stayed on the lounge chair, almost paralysed, not knowing what to do or expect.

The pain was in my lower abdomen and very intense. I dragged myself to the toilet and then, with an expulsive push, I felt a release.

All these clots and blood came pouring out. I grabbed a pad to put between my legs as the blood kept coming.

"Take me to the medical centre," I called out to Barry. "I think I've had a miscarriage."

"Yes, you have had a miscarriage," Doctor Symes confirmed as we sat in his room. "I will need to do a D & C (dilate & curette) next week," he said as he rang the hospital to book me in.

"Go to the hospital on Monday morning at 7am. You'll need to fast from midnight. They know you're coming, so they'll be expecting you. I'll come up at 8am and take you to theatre to clean out your uterus. You should be able to go home in the afternoon."

He rubbed my stomach and seemed happy with my blood loss. After that, I came home. It was another blow and another disappointment.

'Will I ever have another baby?' I thought.

I was given a contraceptive injection depo provera, apparently to give my body time to recover. My body was very sensitive to the drug and I had no periods or ovulation for over eighteen months. Unable to get pregnant, my misery continued. Despite all the will in the world, my body was rendered incapable.

The anniversary of Shelley's birth arrived. I had cried for most of the morning when Barry came into the lounge where I was.

"Not another year of this," he said. "I can't stand it anymore. I can't put up with another year of you crying all the time."

The words were like a knife in my heart. From then on I was numb and felt nothing. I needed Barry to have another baby. That was what I would use him for and nothing else. I felt nothing for him anymore. He had hurt me so much. He didn't understand my pain and had never helped me in my despair. Saying those words was the last nail in the coffin for my feelings for him. I left the room.

My attention turned to Kelvin. I was with him all day, every day. Even though I still struggled with depression and battled suicidal thoughts, I decided to put everything into him. I bought him pre-school workbooks to do and, even though he was just over two, I started to teach him.

I started to spend more time with him – teaching him, taking him to preschool and buying him educational books and toys. He was going to do well. I always knew that he was a bright little boy. I had known that from the time he was born. He had looked around so intently at the world around him.

He passed his milestones well ahead of a normal toddler. I wanted Kelvin to be educated and to far exceed what Barry and I had achieved. I wanted him to go to university and reach his full potential. He gave me a reason to keep going, even though I still struggled every day.

I began to think about the possibility of doing my nursing training. I wrote to enquire about it. When I got the letter back, it said I would be required to live in Palmerston North, as all the students had to live in at the nurses' home. I would have to do all different shifts at the hospital and be available to go to lectures.

I enquired no further. Barry and I talked about it and realised it would be unworkable, especially with having a toddler. There was no way I could leave him for days on end and expect Mum or Barry's mother to care for him. My dream was once again put on hold. It seemed that it would never come to pass.

'Sometimes things are just not meant to be,' I thought.

Kelvin was nearly four years old when I finally gave up trying to get pregnant and decided to go back to work at the maternity annexe. The place seemed to have a pull on me. I loved my work there and being back again. It was like coming home and I slotted right back in. Everyone was pleased to see me and I started to feel normal and happy again.

Mrs Brunton welcomed me with open arms, as did all the other staff from both maternity and general. The distraction of working and not trying to get pregnant seemed to be what was needed. After a few short months of being back at work, I was pregnant. I was so thrilled to be having another baby and decided to leave work shortly after I found out. I was paranoid I would lose this one too. I hated letting Mrs Brunton down by leaving, but I knew she would understand. I was going to take no chances of losing this one or having another miscarriage. I just wanted to stay at home and grow a baby, no matter how bored I became.

An Angel Arrives

THE NIGHTMARE OF THREE-AND-A-HALF YEARS ago seemed to be happening all over again when I ended up going into hospital for bed rest at 38 weeks pregnant. This time it was only two weeks before my due date when I ended up in the same antenatal room I had been in with Shelley. It felt like I was reliving the events of Shelley's birth all over again. Complete bed rest again for pre-eclampsia. Not a lot of fun, but I didn't care. I would do anything to hold a baby in my arms.

Doctor Symes came around the next day. "Are you feeling alright about this?" he said. I gathered he meant, "Are you ok that we are back here again?"

I lied and said, "Yes, I'm ok."

All the time, I was feeling dread at the thought of something wrong happening again. I put on a brave face. On one hand, I was afraid that the nightmare was happening again, but then, on the other hand, I was excited that I was near the end. Very soon I would have the baby I had longed for. It had been a long, emotional road over the past three-and-a-half years and, even now, I had very mixed emotions. This pregnancy had given me hope for the future. Once I had a baby in my arms, I might even be the happy, carefree person I used to be.

So for the next two weeks I was looking out at the rose gardens again, having meals brought to me. The highlight of my day was getting visitors, especially when Mum came and brought Kelvin to visit. She had been so faithful in coming up to see me every day and helping out. Barry came in the evenings. After that, he would go and get Kelvin and take him home for the night, then he would drop him back at Mum's or his mother's in the morning. I had regular blood pressure checks, palpation of my abdomen and listening to the baby's heartbeat. About four times a day the sisters would come in and check on the baby and me.

I had been in hospital for two weeks when Doctor Symes came into my room.

"I think we will induce you tomorrow. I don't want to wait any longer. Everything is good right now and I don't want to wait till the placenta starts deteriorating," he said. "I will come in tomorrow and break your waters in theatre."

I had been down this road twice before and felt anxious about it. I didn't sleep at all that night, but just lay awake thinking of the next morning and how was it going to be.

With fear and anxiety I thought, 'At last, not long now.' Was it going to be the birth of a beautiful, healthy baby, or was it going to be like last time, with all my dreams being shattered? I couldn't conceive the latter. How would I ever be able to carry on?

The next day I was taken into theatre and was put into the familiar legs-up-in-the-lithotomy position. I was given some pethidine again and so felt quite relaxed when he put his hand up my vagina, used the amnihook to find the cervix, and water gushed out. I was then wheeled back to my room to await the much anticipated contractions.

"Sit up as much as possible," Sister Drury said. "Let the water drain out."

The day dragged, but nothing happened. At the end of the day I had no contractions and there was no sign of me going into labour. It did seem like déjà vu and I tried not to think about it. One thing I knew was that this baby was going to be born in the next day or so, one way or another – whether it was going to be healthy or not was out of my hands.

Nothing happened all day, not even one contraction, so I was surprised when I woke in the middle of the night feeling painful tightenings. I lay there for quite a while thinking, 'Is this it or not?' I rang the bell after realising I was indeed contracting. Sister Shannon, who was on for that night, came in when I rang the bell. She felt my abdomen and listened to the baby's heartbeat.

"Looks as if you might be going into labour," she said. "The baby's heart is fine, so we will just see how you progress and if you get into proper labour or not."

With that, she left the room and I tried to settle back to sleep.

I continued to contract regularly, with some becoming quite intense. In the dark, I was quietly labouring and coping well. I never rang the bell again, just kept contracting and breathing through them. I was lying on my side, breathing through each contraction as it came. I had no idea of the time. I must have lain there for a couple of hours, when I suddenly felt something wet between my legs.

The contractions were strong by this stage and with each one I had to concentrate on my breathing. I rang the bell as the contractions kept coming and I felt something coming out of my vagina. I put my hands down there as Sister Shannon came into the room and turned the light on. I brought my hand up to look at what it was and my hand was covered in a black, thick tar.

"Is that me?" I said to Sister Shannon, not realizing what I was seeing.

"It's meconium," she said and with that disappeared.

After a few minutes she was back and frantically trying to get the bed out of the room. She quickly opened the doors and pulled the bed out all on her own, so that she could wheel it down the corridor.

My contractions were very intense and I started to feel like I wanted to push. There was an air of urgency and panic as she frantically tried to get the bed down the corridor and through the doors.

"I'm in so much pain," I called out "I want some pethidine. Please can I have some pethidine?"

The lights were on in the theatre room and she pulled me onto the theatre bed then took the other bed out. All I could hear was banging and crashing of doors and beds. Everything seemed to be happening so fast.

"Come down to the end of the bed, Julie," she said as she tried to help me move. I could sense panic in her voice. I was lying on my back and wriggled down as far as I could.

"That's great," she said as she took my legs and started to put them up in the metal stirrups, which were at each side if the bed.

Next thing I heard Doctor Symes outside the theatre door getting his gumboots on. There was no mistaking that cough.

"Oh no," I called as the next contraction came. I felt my stomach rise and intense pain in my lower abdomen.

I breathed through as best I could.

"Can I have some pain relief?" was all I could say when it finished.

"No, it's too late for that," she said. "You can have some gas." And with that, she thrust the tube into my hand.

Sister Shannon then went over and started opening packs and instruments.

"Open some forceps and get me some obstetric cream," I heard Doctor Symes say. "It looks as if this baby is breech," he said.

With that, I gave an almighty push. I could feel the baby coming. I just kept panting and breathing. Whenever a contraction came, I had an almighty urge to push.

"It is coming fast," he kept saying to Sister Shannon. I continued to feel like pushing and just closed my eyes and went with it. I was lying on my back and looking at the ceiling with my legs spread out and my bottom perched at the end of the narrow bed that I lay on. I kept pushing with every contraction. It seemed to be happening so fast.

"It is breech alright. Get me that towel." I heard him say.

I kept pushing as each contraction came.

"Look, the baby is coming down nicely." He said reassuringly to Sister Shannon.

"Can I have the Wrigley's forceps on the trolley?" I heard him say.

I just closed my eyes and breathed on the gas. The next contraction came and I felt the excruciating pain of metal instruments being put up inside me and screamed out in pain. I felt like I was being ripped open as the instruments were put up inside me and onto the baby's head. With a pull on the head and my final scream, I felt relief as the head was released from my body.

I heard the hearty cry of a baby. "You have a girl," Doctor Symes said.

It was 3:10 in the morning, only three hours after I had rung the bell the first time. It had been quick labour and an undiagnosed breech birth.

The baby kept crying as Sister Shannon handed her to me. The elation was overwhelming. After all the suffering of the past three-and-a-half years, I had a baby girl. I was so excited and thrilled.

"This is the best day of my life," I said and I believed that it was.

She was a healthy little girl. She was so lovely and pink with beautiful, golden hair. I fell in love with her as I held her in my arms – the arms that had been empty for so long.

I was on the bed being wheeled back when I came into the corridor and saw Barry standing with a grin from ear to ear. There was no silence from the labour room this time. No mistaking the lusty cry of a healthy baby.

"What did we have?" He asked as he followed the bed.

"You have a beautiful baby daughter," Sister Shannon said, beating me to giving the good news. She was in my arms and, for a lovely time, Barry and I were just left to gaze at her in awe and wonder.

We were both so elated that all was well. I lay her on the bed and started unwrapping her. Yes, all her fingers, toes, arms and legs were fine. She was a pale-skinned, pink baby with light, golden hair down to the nape of her neck. We pondered what would we call her. Now that we had met her, we thought about what suited her, what name she looked like.

Barry stayed with me for about an hour and then had to go home to bed. Sister Shannon came and took the little one back to the nursery. Rules had started to relax. Rooming in was starting to come in, but still at the discretion of the staff. Obviously Sister Shannon wanted me to go back to sleep.

As I heard one of the women get up to feed her baby, I called out, "I've had a girl. My baby is born and she is ok. She is ok!" I called out.

Hoping I would be heard, I was crying now out of sheer relief and joy. I felt as if I would never come down from the cloud I was on. I stayed awake, even though I had been instructed to go back to sleep. That was never going to happen. No way was I going back to sleep. I just stayed awake until day break. My excitement and joy was so great that I felt like my heart would burst. It was so great having a baby at last and it was such a bonus that it was a little girl. It was more than I had dared to dream for.

When Barry came the next day, we discussed her name.

"What do you think?" I asked. "I was wondering about Angela, since she is like an angel. And she looks like an angel, don't you think?"

"Yes, that sounds nice. Did you still think Mary for the second name?" Mary was Barry's sister's name. So her name was decided on – Angela Mary Watson. She was such a placid baby and latched onto the breast no problem. I was going to enjoy every part of mothering her and breastfeed as long as I could, I thought.

Breastfeeding went well with Angela and was a very different experience from when I breastfed Kelvin. I was able to feed her when she was awake and hungry. The babies were still kept in the nursery overnight, but they were by their mothers' beds during the day.

The thrill of Angela's birth was overwhelming. I never thought at the time, though, that having a vaginal breech birth could be hazardous. It was only years later that I realised the outcome could have been very different.

Is She Blind?

THE THREE-AND-A-HALF YEARS FROM SHELLEY's death to Angela's birth had been a difficult time. Kelvin and the hope of having another baby had given me the will to keep going.

With the birth of our new baby, came new hope and a sense that the dark days were over. We doted on our new baby and were overjoyed to have her. It was back to the routine of caring for a newborn baby – breastfeeding, getting up in the night for feeds, and all the extra washing of nappies and baby clothes. Breastfeeding was a breeze compared to last time and Angela was a content and happy baby. I was so tired from all the extra work that a baby brings, but I was blissfully happy. I enjoyed every minute. She was due for her check-up at six weeks old, so I took her along to the medical centre. I hadn't noticed anything wrong, so I was taken aback when Doctor Symes noticed that she could not follow his finger when he moved it across in front of her eyes.

"I think she is blind," he said. He kept trying to get her to respond to his finger by moving it from one eye to the other. "She should be able to follow my finger at this age."

"What?" I said. "Blind. No, she can't be blind." I was stunned, numb and couldn't believe what I was hearing.

"Bring her back in a month. I'll check her again and refer her to an eye specialist if I still have concerns. It is difficult when they are so young, so try not to worry too much." Doctor Symes tried to reassure me, but the look on his face said it all.

I left the doctors' surgery in a dazed state, wondering what this would all mean. I couldn't believe that the amazing high of the past six weeks had now been replaced by this devastating news. The bubble had burst. Could it be that, after all we had been through, we were facing bringing up a child who was, indeed, blind? It was inconceivable that this beautiful baby, who I had longed for, might not be able to see and have a normal life.

As she was so young, there was nothing that could be done. We just had to wait and see. We started watching her every move intently, observing whether she was responding to what was happening around her and looking for signs that she could see.

We tried to carry on as normal, minding our little daughter and enjoying every minute that we had with her. She was smiling, but it was a bit later than normal. Was she smiling in response to what she could see, or was she smiling in response to the voices she heard?

It was so hard to tell when she couldn't speak. We continued to play the waiting game and just enjoyed having her as part of our family. No matter what the outcome, we loved her. We had waited so long for her that we felt we would be able to handle whatever the verdict was. She was very content and easy to look after, hardly ever crying or making a fuss.

When Angela was six months old, an opportunity came for a weekend away at the bach. Dad rang up.

"Would you like to come out to the coast this weekend? Mum and I thought we would go out on Friday night. We are taking Grandad as well."

It was a welcome break and we jumped at the chance. We seemed to be spending less and less time at the beach recently. Barry had joined the fire brigade, so he wanted to be in town a lot of the time in case there was a fire.

We arrived at the bach on Friday night, unpacked all our gear and, after having something to eat, fell into bed. The sound of the waves crashing in the distance helped me drift off to sleep. I woke with the sun streaming into the bedroom window. The window faced the sea and the rising sun. I could hear the men in the living area, laughing and talking. Dad, Grandad and Barry put the crayfish pots out before the sun came up. They had come back and were now preparing breakfast.

"Who wants a cooked breakfast?" Grandad called out to Mum and me as we lay in bed enjoying the chance to lie in.

"Yes, please," I called as I got out of my bunk bed and came into the living area.

Grandad was the self-appointed cook while out at the bach. He loved to cook, especially the seafood we would catch. Paua fritters and crayfish were his specialty.

Kelvin had already got up and Angela was still asleep, as I had fed her earlier.

"Gorgeous, isn't it?" I said as I looked out to sea. The sun had risen and was casting a yellow reflection on the blue sea below. The bach was on a hill. From the living area, we had a panoramic view of the sea, which stretched from Cape Turn Again to Castlepoint, including the lighthouse in the distance.

'What a paradise,' I thought as I marvelled at the view in front of me.

The bach was a small house, consisting of a large living and dining area in the middle, which went from the back of the house to the large windows and double doors in the front that faced the sea. Off the living area, there were two bedrooms, one on either side. Also off the living room, was the bathroom and, opposite the bathroom on the other side of the living area, was the kitchen, which led to an outside door. The toilet was outside and was a long drop. It was a few years before an inside toilet was put in the bathroom.

Grandad set about cooking us bacon and eggs for breakfast. He loved it here and took every opportunity to come out with Mum and Dad.

"Come and get it," he called as the breakfast was put on the table.

"Be back in a minute," I said as I rushed outside to the loo.

I was busting. I had put off going in the night as I had a healthy fear of possums and they had a habit of being around at night. My sister had one jump on her from the toilet roof once, and, from then on, I would try and wait until the morning to go to the toilet to avoid a similar encounter.

Breakfast was over and the dishes were done. The crayfish pots were out in the sea until the evening. Fishing and catching crayfish depended on the tides, which Dad studied meticulously. Once the crayfish pots were in the sea, Dad would often go and surf cast off the large rocks that were further along the coastline in a bid to catch that elusive snapper. He would find a spot nestled amongst the rocks where he could put his line out and be safe from the pounding surf below.

Later on in the morning, Barry and I decided to take the kids down to the water's edge in front of the bach and let Kelvin play in the rock pools. When the tide was out, the sharp rocks were visible and, all the way out to the breaker line, pools of water were left.

Even though there was no beach at Mataikona, the rock pools made excellent paddling pools when the tide was out. They were safe with the natural barrier of the rocks surrounding them. A lot of the pools near the high tide mark had sandy bottoms and the water was only knee deep, so it was ideal for a five year old to have a splash.

The day was lovely. There was no wind and the sun was shining. We thought it was a perfect chance to take both the kids down to the sea before Angela was due to have her morning nap. The rock pools were just in front of the bach. We crossed the road and walked along the narrow track that went through the rushes and flax bushes to the stones at the edge of the rocks. The breaker line was in the distance, at the end of the jagged rocks that stretched about 30 metres out.

Kelvin ran ahead with a bucket and spade in hand, ready to play in the pools. We followed, with Barry carrying Angela. As we approached the water's edge, Angela started screaming and crawling up Barry's shirt like a wild animal. She was desperately trying to get away and we realised that the sound of the sea and the roar of the waves was causing her to scream in fear. It was obvious that she couldn't see what was causing the roar. The sound of the crashing waves terrified her.

We could hardly hold her and it took the two of us to prevent her from falling to the stones below.

"Come on, Kelvin. We have to go back," I said, grabbing his hand.

I was shaking with anxiety as we hurriedly made our way back through the rushes, over the road and back to the bach. I had never thought that the sound of the sea would sound so scary to someone who couldn't see very well. We never took her down to the sea again until she was older, when we could explain what the roar of the sea was and the sound of the crashing waves.

Angela seemed slow to venture out and explore the world around her. She was happy to just sit on the floor and play with the toys placed around her.

"She can't see normally, but to what extent I am not sure," Doctor Bolton told us when we took Angela to her at a year old. "It is very difficult when she can't tell us what she can see. It might be a while before we can accurately find out the extent to which she can see or not. We just have to give it a bit more time. In the meantime, though, whenever you take her outside or in the sun, you'll have to protect her eyes."

Angela was sixteen months old when she finally took her first steps and began to walk. I was beginning to think we were going to have to carry her around forever.

We were going back to the eye specialist, Doctor Bolton, every six months but, between visits, there was nothing much we could do. It was too soon to test her eyesight properly and to get a correct diagnosis. We would have to wait until Angela was two years old before we would learn more.

"Angela has albinism," Doctor Bolton said. "Her eye is shaped like a football and not round like most people's eyes. She also has no pigment in her skin and no protection from the sun. When she goes in the sun, she will need to have eye protection and you must be careful not to expose her skin, as she will burn very easily. Normally people with albinism have very poor eyesight and it will take a few more visits and tests to determine how bad her eyesight is, but we will fit her with glasses now to help her see better."

Once Angela had glasses fitted at the age of two, she was a different child and she was much more adventurous. She never took her glasses off, as she wanted to take in her surroundings and the new world that had opened up to her.

Genetic counselling followed and the condition was explained to us. There was a one-in-four chance that we would have another baby with albinism, as both Barry and I had a recessive gene carrying albinism. We were determined that Angela would be treated normally and not be wrapped in cotton wool. We didn't bring attention to her condition, so she adapted and coped with it as she grew up.

She was registered with the blind foundation, which gave her support in her schooling. Her eyesight did limit her from playing some sports, especially team sports, but she loved swimming and did ballet until the age of eight.

Schoolwork was a challenge but, despite the obstacles, she did well. Mostly her eyesight didn't stop her from doing anything she wanted. Obtaining her driver's licence, however, was something she would always have to live without.

A Light Switched On

ANGELA WAS ABOUT A YEAR old when I went back to work at Pahiatua Hospital. I would have liked to be a stay-at-home mum and be content with domestic duties, but I was not wired that way and always felt the need to work. I got bored and depressed when I was at home for any length of time, and always felt the need to work and be around other people. I only worked part time so I could balance both home and my job with the help of both sets of parents, who would mind the children when needed. Doing shift work was always a juggle with children but, with their help, we seemed to manage it.

Since Shelley's birth and even after the birth of Angela, depression was never far away. It never seemed to completely leave me. It was as if my soul had been scarred and the damage could never be repaired. I could never go back to the person I once was. The carefree person I once was had been replaced by someone who was depressed and anxious. My relationship with Barry had improved, but I still resented the fact that he had not been there when I needed him. I would bring it up on a regular basis, whenever we had a disagreement or argument.

"You will never forgive me," he used to say. Another pet saying was, "I am not a mind reader," when I would tell him of his shortfalls.

I struggled with depression, loneliness and self-doubt and would take it out on him. I blamed him for everything. I felt I had no friends and that it was his fault. I blamed him for my unhappiness because he didn't understand how I felt and could never meet my emotional needs. Barry was never very social and I needed to be around people, so I blamed our lack of social contact on him.

I carried on. Most of the time that I was working I felt fine but, when I had time to think or was alone, the feelings returned. I could never shake it off. It didn't matter how Barry was towards me. I always remembered that he wasn't there for me when I needed him the most.

What was done could never be undone. He would listen to me and never get angry, just frustrated that I always felt this way and that I could never seem to move on or forgive him. I would always bring it up. It was like an old recording that I would play whenever we were having an argument.

I started to wonder where Shelley was and if she was in heaven, or even if there was a heaven. I had never thought about such things at all before, but the loss of Shelley left me wondering what had happened to her and if I would ever see her. I found it hard to accept that she was gone forever. I started looking for some hope in my life. As a child, I went to Sunday school, like most kids did in the 1960s, so I was drawn back to the church where I had attended Sunday school. I wanted to find some hope that Shelley was in heaven and that heaven existed. I wanted to believe that God did exist, that there was a future and life after death.

I went along to the little Presbyterian Church I had attended as a child and where we got married. I found that it had changed a lot.

There were people with guitars playing upbeat music and singing modern songs rather than the old hymns that I remembered. It all seemed to be very happy-clappy and I enjoyed the service very much.

I started going to church sometimes and gradually went more and more, until I was going every Sunday morning that I could.

I kept wondering about God and his existence. I decided to pray and see if any of my prayers would be answered.

"God, if you are real, show yourself to me. If you are there, come and help me," I would pray.

As well as going as often as I could on Sunday mornings, I also started attending a home group on Wednesday nights. I would pray and ask God for things and read the Bible that I had been given. I would read and pray secretly in the bedroom, concealing what I was doing from Barry. He saw me, though, and said to come into the lounge and read there. I sheepishly took the Bible into the living room, embarrassed about what I was doing.

No one in our family was religious and it was like there was a stigma attached to anyone I knew who did have a faith. Not that I knew very many people who did believe in God. My grandfather was an atheist and his favourite pastime was to argue with the Jehovah's Witnesses when they came to the door. He loved to bail them up in the doorway, not letting them escape until he had, in his eyes at least, won the argument with them.

My life had changed focus and I was intent on finding out the truth. I followed my heart and not my head in all this. If God revealed Himself to me, then I would believe and give it my all. Certainly I started to feel more peaceful and a sense that I was embarking on an adventure. That I was going to find the secret to life itself, which seemed to be hidden from most people.

I became more excited as prayers started to be answered. The grass became greener and the sky bluer. The flowers had more colour and I became amazed at the world around me. I was seeing the beauty of creation, the power of the sun and sea. I would wake up every morning and look out the window, seeing beauty that I had never noticed before.

It was as if God was bringing my attention to the beauty and the detail of everything in the world. From the grass and the flowers, to the vast animal kingdom. The variety of insects, animals and humans in the world.

Every time I went to church and started to sing, I felt his presence with me, as if he was standing beside me. I continued to read the Bible with an insatiable hunger and the words seemed to come alive. I started to believe every word that was written in it and life began to make sense.

Christmas carols and hymns that I had known all my life seemed to have meaning now, as the words spoke of the truth I was discovering. They were not just words that were sung. The real meaning contained in the songs gave them life.

Gradually, my belief in the words written in the Bible strengthened. It was revealed to me that Jesus Christ had come, lived and died for mankind. That He was the Saviour of the world. That if I gave my life and heart to Him, I would not only have life here on Earth. When I died, I would live for eternity with Him.

I was baptised on Easter Sunday 1982 and committed my life to being a Christian. My life started to change as I prayed and was guided by Him, believing that God wanted the best for me and loved me. It was as if I had embarked on an adventure. I did not know where it would lead and it was exciting, full of hope and expectation.

I started to believe that, no matter what happened in my life, God was with me and wanted the best for me. That I could trust Him and that He had a plan for me, which was good because He loved me.

I slowly began to forgive Barry and started to look more positively towards the future. I realised that if we were to have any future together and if we were going to stay married to each other, that I needed to forgive him and move on. That nothing would change what had happened in the past and we had to forgive each other. We had both been punished enough.

A Gift Given

Barry and I came to the decision not to have any more children after Angela was born. The emotional toil had been great and I felt like I couldn't take any more. As we now had a son and a daughter, we decided that our family was complete. There was nearly five years between Kelvin and Angela and, even though there was normal sibling rivalry, mostly they got on well.

I still struggled at times with depression, even with my new-found faith, but I was better than I had been, and Barry and I were happy. Slowly I was healing and, with every passing year, the pain became less. Barry had mellowed so much. He just wanted me to be happy and would do anything for me. He had also become a Christian, a few months after me, and life was good. So often I had wanted to leave him in the earlier years, but now I was pleased I had stuck with it and I'm sure he felt the same way. It had been tough for both of us.

We were in our first house for eight years before we bought Barry's parents' lifestyle block, as they had moved to a larger property. Barry was very keen to move to his parents' place, where he had grown up. I was less enthusiastic but, in the end, reluctantly moved. I loved our first home and had become quite emotionally attached to it, but I conceded that there was going to be more room for the kids to run around if we had some land. We could have hens, sheep and cattle at the new place, as well as a large garden to grow all our own vegetables. The house was not a patch on our first home and Barry set about doing it up as soon as we moved in. In six months he had completely redecorated the whole house.

On the farm, we had hens for eggs, a massive garden, and sheep and beef for our own use. There was a large row of sheds at the back of the farm, which were full of machinery, tractors, equipment and anything and everything you would need on a farm – or not need, as the case may be. Barry's father left it all when he moved. Nothing was thrown out, just in case it might be needed.

From the time Angela was a year old, I was back working at the hospital. It was what I knew and what was comfortable. Now, though, I worked in both the maternity ward and general ward. There were more enrolled nurses working and, since I was not trained, I had to work where I was needed, not where I preferred.

When Angela was five years old, I heard that a local retail dress shop was on the market and, following a lot of discussion, Barry and I decided to buy it and that I would run it. My Aunty Joyce, who was Mum's sister, was working in the shop already and she was pleased when we bought it, as we would work together. My Aunty and I had always got on well and she had so much experience in clothes and retail that I knew it would work.

During this time, after about five years on the farm, Barry and I decided to sell the land and move into town. Living on the farm gave us a great lifestyle but it did have its downside. Having the animals meant we couldn't just go away whenever we felt like it. Our times of going out to the bach had become less frequent as we had to plan for someone to feed and mind the animals. Moving back into town would make it easier to get away.

We bought a large split-level property with four bedrooms, a dining/lounge area and a separate lounge adjacent to the front door and entrance hall. It was a very spacious house and the grounds were large, with plenty of lawns and gardens. We moved into 40 Princess Street, only a block from Mum and Dad's house, in 1984.

I had been in the shop for nearly four years when a thought came to me that I had been on the contraceptive pill for eight years. For some reason, this started to concern me and I decided that being on the pill for so long couldn't be good for my body. I came to the conclusion that it was time I came off the pill for a time to give my body a break. Without much thought, I stopped taking the pill. My mind was so preoccupied with running the shop that I gave no thought that I might become pregnant.

"Well, often these babies that are unplanned are the most cherished of all," Doctor Symes said when the pregnancy test came back positive.

The news could not have come during a more untimely period. I was running a shop that was hardly making any money and I couldn't afford to have someone running it full-time. Aunty Joyce was amazing, but I couldn't ask her to do more than what she was already doing.

I would wake up in the middle of the night worried about how it was going to work and how I was going to run the shop with a little baby. We had nothing for the baby, as all the baby furniture and clothes had long gone. It was like having our first baby again. I felt completely vulnerable and all I could do was to pray for a solution.

For seven months, I prayed every day to sell the shop and, in the end, gave up as nothing was happening.

"Well, God, if you want me to have the shop and have a baby out the back while I'm working in it, so be it," I told God in my frustration.

It was about a week later when a woman came in off the street and enquired about buying the shop. I couldn't believe it and felt such a relief when the shop finally sold and the burden was lifted from me. The deal went through quickly and I was home about four weeks before Elizabeth was born. I was amazed to think that at the last minute, my prayers had been answered. It was just in the nick of time.

I chose to have an obstetrician look after me with this baby, as I was reluctant to risk any unforeseen circumstances after my checkered obstetric history. Even though I still had pre-elampsia, I was induced early and avoided being admitted for bed rest.

Our surprise baby was born on Christmas Eve 1986, after a six-hour labour. Both Barry and I felt so blessed when she arrived. She was beautiful and weighed 6lb 9oz. It was the first and only birth that Barry attended. After he helped move the bed into the delivery room, he had the door shut behind him and Dawn the midwife said, "You're not going anywhere."

Barry was quietly pleased that he had been present at her birth, although he never admitted it. I noticed though, from the time of her birth, he had a special bond with her and took on the task of bathing her every evening. It was a task I never seemed to get to do, but I was happy that Barry was more involved with looking after his daughter.

We named our youngest daughter Elizabeth Jane. The name Elizabeth means gift from God. The whole family loved her, doted on her and played a part in caring for the new baby. Both Angela and Kelvin were old enough to help with caring for their new sister, as well as helping around the house.

I enjoyed being at home for a change and not having to leave the house every morning to go to work in the shop. It wasn't long before we realised that Elizabeth had albinism like her sister. We were not daunted by it, as we knew what was involved because Angela had the same condition.

The whole family loved Elizabeth and she was showered with many gifts following her birth. Because she was born on Christmas Eve, every birthday and Christmas there were loads of presents for Elizabeth. Everyone in the family had a hand in caring for her and was willing to help out. Both Kelvin and Angela would take her for walks and nurse her when she cried. It was as if she had four parents instead of two.

A Flame Ignited

FROM SOON AFTER MUM AND Dad were married, they had lived in Princess Street. It was their home for all their married life and I had lived there for all of my childhood.

Since I had to pass Mum and Dad's house whenever I went to town, I would frequently call in to see them. They were retired now and lived a relaxed life and went on frequent holidays. They both played bowls and Dad played golf. Dad was also an active member of the RSA, as he had been a soldier in World War II and served overseas in Egypt, Italy and Japan. The war had ended while Dad was on the high seas heading for North Africa. His battalion helped for eighteen months in the aftermath of the war. He didn't talk a lot about the war, but he did say that when they went to Hiroshima after the atomic bomb had been dropped, they got out off the train and for as far as the eye could see, the land was flattened, without any signs of life, apart from one solitary tree.

It was lovely having Mum and Dad just down the road when we moved into Princess Street and they would often care for Elizabeth. I enjoyed having a new baby and, even though it was a bit of an adjustment, Elizabeth brought our family incredible pleasure and joy. I would spend my days caring for her, just the two of us, while

Kelvin and Angela were at school and Barry was at work.

I breastfed her for a year and would take her for walks most days. I had worried about having another baby, but it couldn't have been more perfect for our family. Kelvin and Angela enjoyed her as much as Barry and I did.

By the time Elizabeth was three, Kelvin had enrolled at Massey University for the following year and Angela was in her first year of secondary school. How the years had flown. It didn't seem that long ago that Kelvin was a baby, and now he was leaving home and going to make his own way in the world.

It was lovely being at home, but I needed to work. I always had the need to feel that I was contributing in some way. The hospital seemed to be my only choice. I had loved working in the maternity annexe. Those years were my most enjoyable time at the hospital, but times were changing. Working in maternity was an option that had long gone.

Mrs Brunton had retired now and there was another matron. In fact, a lot of the staff had changed and there were less untrained staff and more registered nurses and enrolled nurses. It was the September school holidays when I started back at the hospital. A new nurse had started whom I had never met.

Sue was only working at the hospital for the school holidays, as she was doing her training to become a registered nurse. I got talking to her at morning tea and my heart leaped as she started to tell me her story. I was amazed at how similar our lives were. She had also married young and had five children. She had always wanted to train as a registered nurse but had not had the opportunity until now.

"I just felt it was my time," she said. "It is now or never, since it's never going to perfect timing for our children. If you wait till they are grown up and have left home, it is almost too late. This is my first year and I love it. It's not easy, though, and I have to spend all my spare time studying. When I'm home, I have to do assignments and study. Plus running a home and caring for the children. I have no free time at all."

I listened intently to her story, which seemed so similar to my own. I became excited and hope started to rise within me. Maybe the door to my dream was not yet closed after all.

"I've always wanted to train, but the opportunity was never there. I have given up on ever being able to do it," I said to her. "I thought the door for me was well closed. Are they taking women in their late 30s and not just people out of school?"

"Yes, they are. They're encouraging older people to become trained nurses. There is a lot of support for mature students, with extra tuition if needed. There are a few my age in my class – about four, I think."

For the two weeks of the holidays, she would encourage me every time I saw her at work.

"If I can do it, you can do it," she kept saying.

"If you have support from home and your mum is available to mind Elizabeth, you can do it. You just have to be determined. Set your mind on the goal and just go for it."

I don't think I had ever met anyone like Sue. Her enthusiasm was contagious and, the more I listened to her, the more excited I became that I, too, could do my training.

I certainly didn't want to work as a nurse aide all my life and I could see changes continuing to take place. It wouldn't be too long before there would be no place to care for patients if you were untrained. The only positions I would be able to work in would be domestic duties. The writing was on the wall.

The idea that had birthed within me started to grow as Sue encouraged me. I talked to Barry about the possibility of doing my nursing training and how it would all work.

Barry certainly was not opposed to the idea and was surprisingly supportive. We spent hours talking about how it could be done, including the practicalities of running the home and taking care of Elizabeth.

The brief times I had spent with Sue had rekindled an old flame. She had fanned the smouldering embers that were nearly extinguished. The fire continued to grow within me.

I felt it had been a divine appointment. That God had sent Sue to encourage me and tell me that my dream was still something I could aim for. It was not too late and the opportunity was still there.

Excitement bubbled within me at the possibility. Even the cost of training was taken care of. Barry got a job as a mechanic working for Fonterra, earning as much money as was needed to put me through study. It was as if every obstacle had been blown away.

It was nearing the end of the year. My only hesitation about starting study in the new year was my academic ability. I was excited but also terrified that I would fail – that I would do the training but then not pass the examinations. I had not taken biology at school and it would have been a huge advantage if I had. We decided to delay my training until the following year, and that I would study human biology by correspondence to get a good grounding before I started. Another year wouldn't hurt and by then Elizabeth would nearly be at school, which would make it easier to juggle her care. It would also get me used to studying and I would be able to see if the grey matter was still up to the task of learning. If I started the following year, I would be 37 years old. I was still young enough to get through and have a lot of working life left. Who knows where it could lead.

For the next year, I worked in the general part of the hospital part time and did the human biology course by correspondence. I enjoyed the challenge and passed each stage with no problems. I was surprised at how I adapted to studying again and how interested I was in the subject. When I took the exam at the end of the year, it was like going back in time. I had to go to Tararua College to sit the exam with all the school children.

I filled in the application form, had the interview and was accepted into the Comprehensive Nursing Programme. It was a full-time three year course, which meant travelling over to Palmerston North every day for lectures and practical placements. All the tests and exams would be in Palmerston North as well, so I would have to travel there Monday to Friday.

I was surprisingly nervous about handing my resignation in to the hospital in December 1990. It was as if all my security would be taken away. My secure job would be gone and, if I failed, I would be left with nothing.

The girls gave me a fantastic send off from Pahiatua Hospital. On my last day, they cornered me and chucked me into a physiotherapy pool that was filled with warm water and loads of bubble bath. I was going to miss them a lot and I was going to miss the hospital, which had been such a big part of my life over the years.

Everything was in place for the change in our family life. Well, as much as we could foresee. Both my parents and Barry's parents were happy to help out when they could and would be a backstop if we needed them. A friend from church, Geraldine, offered to mind Elizabeth. She was at home full time and had seven children of her own, so she was only too happy to have Elizabeth. One of her daughters was Elizabeth's age and she thought it would be nice for her daughter to have a playmate. Kelvin was now at university so Barry and Angela would share the cooking and home duties.

I was as prepared as I could be. Passing the human biology course had given me renewed confidence that I could get back into study and learn new information and skills. I had a grounding that I could launch off from and my brain had started to absorb and retain new information.

Before I started study, we went on holiday to New Plymouth in Barry's father's caravan. It was a time of relaxing, roughing it, enjoying the beach and swimming in the sea. We spent hours walking along the beach at nearby Oakura, drinking up the peace before the busy year that lay ahead. Kelvin joined us and we were a family again for a time.

The next week I started at Manawatu Polytechnic. I was nervous as I said goodbye to the family that morning. The weather was perfect – the sun was shining and there wasn't a cloud in the sky. I weaved through the Manawatu Gorge looking at the bush-clad cliffs on the other side of the river. I thought about the fact that I would be driving this road twice a day for the next three years. As I drove intently around all the bends and curves with the sun streaming in the window, the beauty was stunning. I switched the radio on and listened to the music.

The music took away all thoughts of nervousness or anxiety and

I relaxed as I sang. No one could hear me no matter how loud I sang.

'You're going to be my company as I go back and forth every day for the next three years,' I thought to myself. 'This is the beginning of a new life.'

Born for Life

Holidays

It was nearing the end of the second semester. My last placement before the holidays was in a rest home for the elderly in Palmerston North. I had been working there for three weeks but, after today, the holidays would begin. I enjoyed caring for old people again and doing what was familiar.

The routine was very similar to at Pahiatua hospital. I would get the residents up for their showers, dress them in the morning, put them in the lounge where they would sit for most the day and feed some of them their meals and cups of tea. When time permitted, it was nice to talk to the residents who could communicate. They had a lifetime of experiences and some were happy to share them with anyone who would listen.

I was in familiar territory and there was a certain amount of comfort with this placement. I was able to relax a bit and I kept thinking that it wouldn't be long before I was off for two whole weeks. There would be no driving over to Palmerston North every day, no getting up at 5:30am and no getting home after 6pm in the evening. Still, I had put myself down to work at the hospital during the holidays and I had two assignments to hand in.

The year so far had been full on and stressful. There had been lectures and tests to study for in the different subjects we were taught. I spent all my spare time studying or doing assignments. I wasn't familiar with computers, so I would write the assignment out in longhand and then Barry would type it up and print it out. He had pushed to buy a computer a long time before, as he wanted to keep up with changing technology. I was less enthusiastic, but conceded that before long computers would be part of all of our lives and nothing much would be done without them.

It would be another year before I would be comfortable with the computer and able to do it all myself. I started thinking about what my break would be like. I had loads of work at home to do. My full-time study meant that the house only got a quick going over once a week and it was becoming a struggle to keep on top of the housework.

I had to turn a blind eye to some of it, as there just wasn't enough time to do everything. I kept reminding myself that there was a bigger goal I was aiming for here. As for the housework, well, so long as the basics were done. We were all pitching in and it wasn't that bad really.

I had been sick with the flu twice recently but I just boxed on, pushing myself to carry on since I could not afford to take time out. If I took time off, I might fall behind and there was no way I was risking that. Not after all the sacrifices the family and I had made.

Barry was holding down a job that required him to be on call in the weekends. He was working long hours to get me through study and typing up all my assignments at night, so he was flat out as well. Angela had to cook the evening meal and do some of the housework after school. I hoped all this juggling for the next three years would be worth it and that it wouldn't all explode in our faces. I still felt like I should work in the holidays. I had given up my job at the hospital to do this study and I felt like I needed to contribute financially.

I got home on the Friday afternoon, relieved to be on break, but knowing I had work in the morning and two assignments to complete by the end of the holidays. I still felt unwell from the flu, but I had some medicine from the chemist that seemed to be working, so I wasn't as sick as I had been. Paracetamol would help if I kept taking it regularly and hopefully I would get a good night's sleep before work in the morning.

When I got back into town, I pulled up into Geraldine's driveway to pick up Elizabeth. Lizzie was always thrilled to see me and came running out to greet me. I shut the car door and Lizzie took my hand as I walked down the driveway, onto the deck and into the kitchen. Geraldine was at the bench reading the newspaper.

"Have you got time to have a cuppa? The jug has just boiled." Geraldine said as I came up the steps.

Geraldine was always ready to make a cuppa for me when I came to pick up Lizzie. Most of the time I couldn't stop, but today it was nice to sit down and have a catch up.

"Lizzie fell over and hurt her knee when they were playing out the back earlier. She cried and cried and kept asking for you. 'I want my Mummy. She's a nurse,'" Geraldine said as she got the cups down.

"Was she ok? Did it take her long to calm down? I feel so guilty that I'm not here for her, especially when she needs me. Thanks so much for looking after her. I'm so grateful."

How sweet, I thought, that my baby still wanted me when she was hurting. Kids are so loving and forgiving. Lizzie didn't hold it against me that I wasn't there in her time of need, but she thought

I would know how to fix her skinned knee. Guilt was something I battled with. Would all this be worth it in the end? Was it worth all this stress and upheaval that the family was going through? I was hardly ever there and, when I was there, I was studying, trying to learn everything I needed to.

"Look, Deborah loves having her to play with and they are great friends. She fits in so well. It didn't take long for her to get over her fall and she was playing again in no time."

It was nice to stop and chat for a bit after a hectic week. It was a luxury I often missed out on. I was thankful for a sit down and a catch up before heading home.

Without Geraldine's support and help looking after Lizzie, I doubted I would be able to take on such a commitment. She was amazing at looking after Lizzie while I was studying. She took Lizzie back and forth to kindergarten every day and looked after her until Barry, Angela or I could pick her up.

The reprieve was short-lived and, the minute I was home, dinner had to be prepared.

'It's just a case of being super organised and keeping ahead of everything,' I thought.

The grocery list was on the bench. I went around the house jotting down everything we needed. Barry would go and get the groceries when he got home.

Fitting the basics in like buying the groceries, cleaning the house, changing the sheets and doing the washing was difficult. It was a combined effort from everyone to keep the household running and the house in reasonable order, without things getting behind.

The alarm went the next morning and I dragged myself out

of bed. The flu symptoms had returned and I could hardly lift my head off the pillow, but I was rostered on to work. I forced myself to go through the motions of getting dressed and ready for work. Angela could look after Elizabeth while I wasn't there. It worked out well having a built-in babysitter. It was a real advantage having the children so spread out, even though it wasn't planned that way at all.

I downed some more paracetamol with breakfast and tried to shake off my blinding headache and feelings of listlessness and tiredness. My body just wanted to get back in that bed and have some more rest.

'I'm sure I'll be right when I get there,' I thought.

Angela had her day with Elizabeth planned. I would be home in the afternoon to take over, so that she could do her own thing and go and see her friends.

I arrived at work and went into the general office where the morning shift gathered for handover. There was barely enough room and we all huddled in the office as handover was given by the night sister. At the end of handover, we were allocated the patients we had to care for during the morning.

I was given the two four-bedded rooms in the men's ward. It was a heavy load and, even though we helped each other with the showering and lifting, it was not easy. The shift was physically and emotionally exhausting. By the end of the shift, I could barely drag myself around. I was cold one minute and hot the next, so I conceded defeat and said I wouldn't be in tomorrow. I went home and lay on the couch for the evening but I was no better in the morning. By the end of the weekend, I was still unwell and spending most of the day in bed sleeping.

"I think you shouldn't work these holidays," Barry said that night. "It's just too much and I don't think you are well enough. You need to get better in the next two weeks before you go back to tech."

"I know and I have those assignments hanging over me as well. I need to do them, as the deadline is when we go back after the holidays. I'll ring the hospital in the morning and say I am not able to work these holidays. I think that is the best decision. Then I might be well again by the time I'm due to go back to tech."

I needed to get on top of the sickness that had been plaguing me for the past few weeks. I just couldn't seem to get well, so I needed to rest as much as I could.

I spent the next few days huddled by the fire in a blanket nursing myself, relieved that some of the pressure was off and I could try and rest. I still had the assignments to do, but at least now I had more time to do them. I took it easy over the next two weeks, pacing myself. I still tried to do as much as I could around the house when I felt well enough. In the evenings I was able to do the assignments that were due and swot for my upcoming microbiology exam.

By the end of the two weeks, the assignments were done and I was as prepared as I could be for my exam. The flu symptoms seemed to have gone and I felt well and ready for the new semester ahead.

The Stroke

I WAS PLEASED TO SEE Gael and the girls when we met up before class on the Monday morning after the holidays. It was exciting to be back. There were six older students and we had got to know each other well. We had a bit of a support network going, as we had all taken on the challenge of study as mature students. We were having our normal cup of coffee before going to the lecture hall. Gael looked at me from across the table and her intent look took me back.

"Are you ok, Julie? You look terrible. Your face."

"Why? What's wrong with it?" I asked.

The others around the table were looking and nodding with concerned looks on their faces.

I got up and quickly went to the bathroom. I didn't like the way everyone was looking at me as if something was really wrong. I went to the bathroom and looked in the mirror. I hardly recognized myself. I looked so unwell. My face was pasty white and the right side of my face looked drooped. I felt an overwhelming wave of lethargy, as if I was finished and couldn't do anything even if I wanted to. Until I saw myself in the mirror I hadn't really thought about how ill I was feeling.

I went back to the girls and sat back down in my chair. "I had better go home. I feel so lousy." The eyes around the table agreed.

"I'll tell Jenny that you're not well and had to go home," Gael said referring to our lecturer. "You drive carefully and take care."

"Ok. I had better go." I got up and started making my way to the door. Gael got up and walked with me to the car.

"Are you sure you'll be alright? Do you think you should get Barry to come and get you?"Gael said.

"No, I'll be alright. I know the road like the back of my hand," I reassured her.

I got in the car and drove out of the car park. I don't remember a lot of the trip home. I was on autopilot as I drove over the windy Pahiatua Track and into the car park where Barry worked. I couldn't bring myself to get out of the car. I just pressed my hand on the horn and didn't take it off until someone came.

"What's up? What's wrong?" Barry said when he eventually came out.

"I need to go to the doctor. I'm sick. I can't do anything. I feel so sick." Barry got into the car, drove me to the medical centre and took me in.

As we sat in the waiting room, one by one the practice nurses came and looked at me. "Shouldn't be too long now," one of them said as we waited in silence.

"Julie Watson." I looked up as Doctor Symes called my name and we followed behind him into his room.

I'm not sure what Doctor Symes thought I had, but he gave me an appointment to see the physiotherapist the next morning and some medication for the nausea that was sweeping over me.

At home, I went straight to bed without dinner and just tried to sleep. All night I had to keep spitting out my saliva, as I couldn't seem to swallow and I choked every time I tried to eat or drink.

"Get me a bowl," I said to Barry, who kept coming in to check on me looking so helpless and concerned.

The saliva would build up and, if I tried to swallow, I would choke, so I had to spit it out into the bowl that was on the floor. I couldn't sleep, since I had to stay awake and keep spitting out the fluid gathering in my mouth. I don't think I could have felt any worse.

'Am I dying?' I thought. The possibility seemed very real.

The next morning Barry took me to Jill Woods, who was the physiotherapist in town. He opened the car door and helped me out, supporting me as we walked to the door.

"Come in," Jill led us into her consulting room. "What is the problem?"

Barry started explaining what had happened. No examination was needed since Jill could see how bad I looked. Without hesitation, she voiced her concern.

"You need to go back to Doctor Symes," she said. "I'll ring the medical centre and get you in. You are very sick and look as if you may have had a stroke."

The words rang in my ears. No, surely not. Only old people, really old people, have strokes. I knew that my grandmother had a stroke before she died and it was only a short time from when she had the stroke to when she passed away. Surely, this was not happening to me?

Barry went grey. He seemed to have aged ten years in the past 24 hours. Nothing more was said. Jill rang the medical centre and we drove there.

I jumped the queue and was in the doctor's room in a few minutes, even though the waiting room was full.

He took my blood pressure and said, "You need to go to Palmerston Hospital. You are not well. I think you may have Guillain-Barre syndrome. You need to have some tests done at the hospital. I'll ring Palmerston North Hospital and organise your admission."

I was in a daze as I was put into the ambulance and taken over to the hospital. Barry followed behind in the car. I was quickly put through the emergency department and before long I was in a hospital bed.

"Get me a bowl or something, I'm going to be sick," I said as a wave of nausea came over me. Barry rushed away to get a bowl as I tried to fight the urge to throw up.

'Could I feel any worse?' I wondered. For the rest of the day, the vomiting continued. Not eating or drinking, just vomiting again and again.

I thought I was attending my own wake when the children and Barry came back that evening. They looked as if their mother had already died as I tried but couldn't really talk to them.

I was overwhelmed with nausea and the feeling of just wanting to curl up and sleep. They sat in silence and periodically talked amongst themselves, with faces that nearly touched the ground. The vomiting that had occurred all day subsided and that night I lay in bed sleeping off and on. My thoughts were of nothing. I just wanted to lie in bed and do nothing. I could hardly respond, apart from yes or no answers, and didn't really care about anything.

Over the next few days, I had examinations and checks from a range of doctors and neurologists, who were investigating what was wrong with me. I was on no medication and it was a wait-and-see game. I was allowed out of bed on the third day and decided to venture out for a walk. I didn't ring for assistance, but slowly got out of bed and made my way down the corridor gingerly holding onto the handrail. Next thing I knew, I was coming to. I was on the cold hospital floor and the nurses were trying to get me up and put me into a wheelchair. I had blacked out and the last thing I remember was slowly walking along the railing that lined the corridor.

It was back to bed rest and another contingent of doctors doing examinations and checks. An MRI scan followed and, yes, I had suffered a stroke, although it was mild and, in time, I should recover fully.

Jenny, one of my lecturers, visited me and her words were words I wished I had heard earlier.

"Listen to your body. It's not a machine and won't be pushed beyond its capabilities," she said. "Just concentrate on getting well and don't think about the study at the moment."

Her words were true. I had been treating my body like a machine and driving it as hard as I could.

I might have heeded that warning if I had heard it before, or maybe I wouldn't have listened. My blood pressure was high and I had kept pushing myself regardless of how I felt and what my body was saying. For weeks it had needed rest. Having the flu three times, one after another, should have been warning enough, but I just kept pushing myself beyond what my body could cope with.

I had learnt a valuable lesson and, if I came out of this and carried on, I promised myself I would not abuse my body again. I would listen when it was telling me to rest. Would I ever be able to have another chance? I wanted to continue studying. Even though it was hard going, it was something that gave me a purpose in life. This was a goal I needed to pursue. My family meant the world to me, but I needed to follow my dream and have no regrets, too.

I wanted and needed the certificate at the end of my study to prove to myself that I could do this and, in time, I knew that without it I wouldn't be able to work in nursing at all. My future in nursing would be at an end without the piece of paper I needed.

If I ever got out of here and things returned to normal, I had to continue with my study. I started working in maternity when I was sixteen years old and fresh out of school. I was now 37 years old and it was my time to accomplish what I had wanted to do since I was ten years old. There was no way I was going to give up now. I could still speak and write. My body and brain seemed to be functioning well enough for me to be able to continue. I just needed to rest and recover.

I was in hospital for two weeks before I was allowed home. I was back studying again three weeks after the stroke. I had a bit to catch up on, but it was not unmanageable. From now on, I was not going to attempt to work at the hospital in the holidays and I was going to listen to my body and rest when I needed to.

Barry decided to do more of the household chores and Angela did as well. It was still a combined effort caring for Elizabeth, who was only four years old when I started my study.

It was a lesson well learnt and I heeded the warning given to me.

"Listen to your body. It is not a machine."

For about a year, my body would be freezing cold on one side and boiling hot on the other, especially when I was in bed. Gradually my face returned to normal without drooping on the right side. I slurred my words initially, but my speech also returned to normal.

The only medication I was put on was a low dose of aspirin, which I was to take daily for the rest of my life. My blood pressure came back down to normal. I had a brush with disaster and came away unscathed. I was thankful that I had learnt a valuable lesson and had been given a second chance.

Born for Life

One More Year

After two-and-a-half years of study, the end was in sight. At the end of the year, I would be a registered nurse at last. What would I do after the end of the year and which area of nursing would I go into? There wasn't a particular area that really pushed my buttons and stood out to me.

I reminisced about the years I had spent working at the maternity annexe and how much I had loved working there. I thoroughly enjoyed the maternity placement I did earlier in the year. The idea of carrying on and studying to be a midwife started to grow. Could it be possible that I could keep studying and do midwifery? I went home that night excited at the prospect.

"What do you think, Barry? I would love to continue and study one more year to be a midwife. I know it is more study, but it is what I love. I want to be with women when they are in labour and have their babies. I want to help women have a lovely birth experience. The only thing I want to do is to be a midwife."

Barry didn't jump at the prospect of me studying for another year, but I could see that he did not discount the idea either. He knew what this would mean. We were near the end of three years of hard slog. As for another year – would the family cope?

After a moment of pondering, he looked at me and said, "Well, I suppose we can survive one more year. Just one more year."

He knew what it meant to me and, without his support, I would never be able to do it.

My heart leapt and I threw my arms around his neck. When I started on this journey, I never thought that I would end up doing midwifery. I started thinking about what would be involved. I still had my nursing exams, assignments and placements to finish before the end of the year. I had to finish and pass the final exams before I could get onto the midwifery programme, but I knew that nothing other than being a midwife would satisfy me.

I had always loved being with women during childbirth and Shelley's birth had made it even more important to me. I never wanted any woman to go through what I went through. I started to sense that what I had experienced in life had meaning. Everything I had been through could and would be used for good.

Yes, I thought, God can even use the death of my baby for good in my life. Even though it seemed like so many years ago, it still brought tears to my eyes when I thought of Shelley's birth and how traumatised I was by it. Despite that, my excitement grew and I knew that this was the path that was meant for me. This is what I wanted to do – be a midwife, help women in labour and be part of the most important time in their lives. One step at a time, though. There was still work to be done. I still had half a year to get through before I would become a registered nurse.

I started investigating what was needed for me to carry on and do midwifery. Colleen, one of my lecturers, was a midwife as well as a lecturer in the nursing programme.

I went to meet her. "What a great idea. You will have to be interviewed and, if you get in, it would mean studying in Wellington for a year."

She explained that the focus of midwifery is continuity of care – looking after women throughout their pregnancy, birth and postnatal periods. She explained the importance of working in the community. You could choose to be an independent midwife – working in the community – or work as a core midwife in the hospital.

She gave me the name of the school in Wellington that I had to apply to and explained the changes that had occurred in New Zealand regarding maternity care.

The Nurses Amendment Act had passed in 1990 and was signed off by the Minister of Health, Helen Clark. The legislation allowed midwives to practice autonomously, caring for woman throughout pregnancy, labour and birth, and then postnatally until the baby was six weeks old.

Midwives could now practice independently in New Zealand and have their own private practice, looking after women without the need of a doctor's input. Midwives were able to write out prescriptions for any medication that women might need during a normal pregnancy and order scans and blood tests. As long as a pregnancy was progressing normally, midwives were able to care for the mother and baby independently. It was only if there were complications that a referral needed to be sent to an obstetrician or, in the case of a sick baby, to a paediatrician.

The emphasis was on the midwife and the woman being in partnership, making decisions together about the care given. It was a model of equal power, rather than of a health professional telling the woman what to do and what would happen to her. Power was now given to women, which was so different from my own experience.

"Thank you so much, Colleen. How do I go about getting an interview?"

"If you contact the Wellington Polytechnic, they will send you an application form and, once you've applied, they will set up an interview for you."

I left her office knowing that I wanted nothing else. It was as if this was what I was born for – it had just taken me years to get there. Nothing else thrilled me as much. The years working with women at Pahiatua Hospital had given me a love of and desire to care for women. I was overcome with joy at the thought that perhaps this might become a reality.

All the paperwork was in for my application to get into the midwifery programme. The appointment had been set for the interview that would determine whether I was suitable to become a midwife.

I attended an interview in Wellington and followed Colleen's advice about how to answer the questions and what was important to get into the programme. I valued her input. Even though I was passionate about midwifery, I wanted to ensure that I came across in the best possible light during the interview.

After the interview, I had to wait and see if I would be accepted into the midwifery programme. Being accepted into the programme not only hinged on my suitability to be a midwife, I also had to pass my final examination to become a registered nurse.

Now that the interview was done, I had to focus on finishing the year – getting the never-ending assignments in and studying for the ongoing assessments and tests.

The third year of study flew by and at the end of the year I sat the final examination. I wept afterwards. All the stress and pressure that had built up over the past three years came out. The exam was so important – what if I failed? I couldn't even think about it. I cried because I was so relieved to be finished, but I was also stressed about the decisions I had made in the exam. Had I answered the questions correctly? I kept going over my answers in my head.

I couldn't do anything more but wait and try and enjoy some time off. There was no more to do. The exam had been sat and the papers submitted. It was now time to relax and enjoy the fact that there was no more study to be done. It was the holidays and Christmas was coming. I wouldn't get my result until mid-January, which was a few weeks away.

The two letters arrived on the same day. The letters with their official logos – one from the Nursing Council and one from the Wellington Polytechnic – contained what the future would be.

As I walked from the letterbox down the driveway with the two letters in my hand, Barry met me at the bottom of the steps.

"What if I have failed after all the work and sacrifice? No, I can't open them. You'll have to," I said holding the letters, afraid of what they might say. I thrust them into his hands, wanting to put my hands over my ears for fear of bad news.

His face said it all as he opened the envelope and took out the letter, "You've passed. It's ok, you can look at it – you've passed."

He then opened the letter from the Wellington Polytechnic and again a smile came across his face.

"You've been accepted into the midwifery programme," he said as he opened the second letter.

A wave of relief flowed over me. It was over and I had passed. I was a registered nurse. I could hardly believe it. All the stress, the hard work, the study and everything the family had gone through had paid off. I had also been accepted into the midwifery programme.

I was ecstatic with relief and so excited. We celebrated that night with a nice meal and a bottle of wine. Everyone was so happy and the phone was red hot as I rang Mum and Dad, Barry's parents, Geraldine and the friends I had made during my three years of study.

Along with me, two other nurses who lived in Palmerston North were accepted into the midwifery programme in Wellington. The Wellington Polytechnic put us in touch with each other and we would meet to organise ourselves for the year ahead. Since the midwifery course didn't start until March, I had time for a break and rest.

It was late January when the phone rang.

"Hi, it's Fi here," said the voice on the end of the phone.

"I am doing the midwifery programme in Wellington this year and wondered if you want to car pool with Lois and me. I have rung Lois and she seems keen. Would you like to meet next week and we can talk about it? Lois is happy to meet at her place if you like."

"That would be great. Just let me know what day suits and I'll come over," I said, eager to get together. It would be great to carpool and have the others to share the time with and encourage each other.

Fi was young, bright and full of life. I already knew Lois because she used to live in Pahiatua. We talked about going to Wellington each week. We had to leave early on Monday morning, attend lectures on Monday and Tuesday and then return on Tuesday night. There were times when we had to spend more time in Wellington, but when we didn't have to be there we would work with independent midwives in Palmerston North. Fi, Lois and I got on well. We took turns taking our cars each week and were great support for each other during the year.

We were booked into the Wellington nurses' home for the time we would be in Wellington each week. The building was old and looked as if it was built in the 19th century. At least there was a lift to take our luggage up to our rooms.

It was very basic and not a place you would want to spend much time. The rooms were small, with a bed along one wall, a dresser at the end of the room and a chair. There was a wooden wardrobe where you could put your clothes and your bag. The kitchen was halfway down the corridor and we had to share it with half the floor. The bathroom was also shared.

There was a lounge at the other end of the corridor, with large windows around the end of the room that let the sunlight in. The panoramic view of Wellington city was spectacular and there were doors that went out to a balcony where you could sit and take in the view.

The three of us spent many evenings out on the balcony having our dinner, looking out and enjoying the view and sounds of the city. The weather was surprisingly settled that year. There wasn't nearly enough wind and rain to live up to Wellington's reputation.

It was a fun time and we supported each other through the lectures, exams and assignments that were constantly due. The three of us had different midwives whom we worked with in Palmerston North. We would recount our experiences and the births we had attended, on the way down to Wellington each week.

My first birth as a student was transforming and confirmed that I had made the right decision. I was encouraged by Sue – the midwife I was working with – to put my hands on her hands and guide this new life into the world. I looked down at the little baby who was kicking and crying, announcing to the world that she had arrived. I was overwhelmed with the miracle of the new life that had just emerged into the world.

"Now, just dry the baby off with this towel and pop the baby onto her mum's chest," Sue said as she lifted up the mother's nightie and exposed her bare chest and breasts.

"If the baby comes out breathing well and is nice and pink, we put the baby skin-to-skin with its mother. It encourages bonding and helps with breastfeeding. If you give the baby a time of uninterrupted skin-to-skin when they are first born, breastfeeding is usually more easily established."

After drying the baby, Sue lifted the baby up onto its mother's chest and put a towel and cuddly blanket on the baby's back.

I watched as the baby lay skin-to-skin and the crying turned to silence. The baby calmed down and became peaceful, seemingly enjoying the warmth and comfort of its mother's bosoms.

'What a beautiful sight,' I thought. 'A mother and baby enjoying their first moments together, bonding with each other and meeting each other for the first time.'

As the year progressed, I delivered many babies, both in the hospital and in people's homes. Some births were normal and straightforward, while other women needed to have a caesarean section. No matter how the baby was born, though, all the births were special. Even if the birth ended up having complications and obstetricians were involved, as a midwife you could make a difference to the woman's experience. No matter what the outcome, you were there for the woman to help her to have an experience that would be positive in her life.

As I worked with different midwives, I learnt different ways of practicing and doing things. Some midwives I worked with only worked in the hospital and were experts at looking after a woman who would sometimes need medical intervention. A woman who needed an epidural for pain relief, or a woman needing an assisted delivery or a caesarean section, could still have a lovely birth experience. Some midwives I worked with only worked in the home, providing homebirths and waterbirths.

Whether the baby was born in the hospital or at home, we visited the women at home postnatally. We would check on the health of mother and baby, help establish breastfeeding and ensure the woman was coping with life and her new baby. When the baby was six weeks old, we would the discharge mother and baby to Plunket. Plunket was set up by Doctor Truby King in 1907 to provide support services for families and ensure babies and children would have a nutritious diet, with the aim of reducing child mortality rates. Plunket nurses would check on the health of children from six weeks to five years of age.

The year flew by and, as we came to sit our final exams, we all had to make a decision about where we would work in our new profession. Whether it was at hospital or in the home, we were there to be with women. I eagerly looked forward to making a difference to the women I would be caring for.

Decision Time

THE GRUELLING FOUR YEARS OF study and the busyness of being a mother, wife and full-time student had come to an end. All of the travelling back and forth was also over. It had taken all the energy I could muster and a lot of patience and commitment from the family, especially Barry who had worked so hard to put me through.

We were over the moon when the results came through and I had passed my midwifery exam at the end of 1994. What a relief after all the hard work. I was now a registered nurse and a registered midwife. There was now the decision of where to work. There was the option of becoming an independent midwife but, after some consideration, I decided I wanted to get some experience in a hospital first. Ultimately my goal was to become an independent midwife, but some hospital experience would be beneficial. I needed to choose a good hospital where I could get the experience that I needed.

Pahiatua Hospital was an option, but birth numbers had dropped so much there that getting the experience I needed would be difficult. In the end, I decided a bigger hospital would be a better choice. Palmerston North Hospital on the other hand, was the main secondary hospital of the region and the largest. A hospital somewhere in between the two would be ideal. I wanted to work in a hospital where I could gain experience and where midwifery was promoted and valued.

Wanganui Hospital was an hour away and seemed to tick all the boxes. The hospital had obstetric and paediatric services, so women and babies were both able to be cared for if there were complications. In addition to the secondary care available, women wanting a natural birth had the option of a waterbirth. Natural birth was much promoted and the hospital had very low medical intervention rates.

The reputation of the hospital was one of a strong midwifery focus.

Barry and I discussed the pros and cons of relocating. It was a big decision to make. Both of us had lived in Pahiatua all our lives and both our sets of parents were still there, alive and well.

They had been so supportive and had helped mind Elizabeth throughout my training. Moving would mean leaving them and going to a town where we knew no one. Kelvin was now married and Angela was doing a polytechnic course in Palmerston North. It was only Elizabeth that would have to move with us. She was eight years old and had good friends at school, but we thought she was young enough to make the adjustment to a new town.

We decided to move to Wanganui. Barry was happy to move and didn't have any problem getting a job as a mechanic in one of the local garages. There was a lot involved, but everything seemed to fall into place. Wanganui Hospital was happy to have a new graduate midwife and I was able to start as soon as possible. Elizabeth was enrolled in school and we put our house in Pahiatua on the market.

By the time we came to move, all was in place, except our house had no prospective buyers, so we had no choice but to rent the house out until it sold. We couldn't afford to buy a house in Wanganui until our house was sold, so we lived in a local caravan park for three weeks until we found a place to rent.

Finally, we found a house that was near the hospital and close to Elizabeth's school. We hoped it wouldn't be long before we would be able to buy a house, but in the meantime renting would have to do. At least now we would have time to look at what area of town we wanted to live.

It was a busy time with us moving, Barry and I settling into a new jobs and Elizabeth adjusting to a new school. We seemed to be blazing a trail back to Pahiatua for different reasons on a regular basis.

We had no sooner moved when Dad had a heart attack. He was hospitalised for a short time, but was soon back to good health. Barry and I travelled over to see him as much as we could and to support Mum. It wasn't long before we felt that we could ease off tripping back to Pahiatua so often.

Barry was able to work from 9am till 3pm, which made it possible for him to mind Elizabeth when she wasn't at school. With me doing shift work, it seemed to be the best solution since we had no family in Wanganui to help look after her. When I worked in the weekends, Barry would take Elizabeth to the library or they would go and see a movie. They were able to have a lot of lovely father and daughter time, just the two of them. Barry was used to helping run the home and had become very domesticated, so all the chores were shared between us.

Wanganui was a lovely place to live and the maternity annexe was a lovely place to work. I soon made some nice friends at church and at the maternity annexe. I started work in the postnatal/antenatal ward and it was a full year before I was rostered to work in delivery suite. I didn't mind where I worked, so long as I was learning and getting experience. Any experience in any area of midwifery was valuable.

After being in Wanganui for nearly a year, we had settled into the town and loved being there. Our house hadn't yet sold, so we patiently waited. In the meantime, we rented a house near one of the major parks and enjoyed going there for walks through the bush and around the lake. It was bliss, like being on permanent holiday.

It was the dead of night in the month of August that same year when Barry and I were woken by the sound of the phone ringing. I ran to answer it, not thinking about who might be ringing in the middle of the night.

"It's Mum. She's died. She's dead."

It took me a few seconds to work out that it was Dad on the end of the phone, frantically telling me that Mum had died.

"The hospital just rang and said that when they went to check on Mum they found her dead."

Dad was crying and distraught and it was hard to hear what he was saying through his distress.

"Ok, Dad. We'll be right over. We'll be as quick as we can. Is there someone you could call to come and be with you until we get there? Do you think you could ring Don and Maureen to come over? It will take us a couple of hours before we get there."

I was referring to Dad's younger brother and his wife, who lived in Pahiatua and were his main support in town.

Dad started to calm a little.

"Do you think you could call in and see Lesley on your way and let her know what has happened? I tried to ring her but I can't get through," Dad said.

"Ok, Dad, We'll be as quick as we can. Do you want us to ring Tony or have you rung him already?"

"No, I'm just going to ring him now."

I turned around to find Barry standing in the doorway of the bedroom.

"Mum's dead," I said walking over to him. I just hugged him trying to take in what I had just heard. Lizzie had also woken and come out to see what was happening.

After gathering our thoughts for a few minutes, we started frantically getting together a few clothes and everything we thought we would need for a few days away. It was too early to ring Lizzie's school or Barry's work. I rang the maternity annexe to let them know what had happened and that I would be away for a few days, probably all week. There was not a lot more we could do in the middle of the night. I was dazed and in disbelief as we drove first to Feilding to let my sister know what had happened and then on to Dad.

I couldn't help but feel guilty and full of regret that I had taken Lizzie to a movie the day before instead of going to visit Mum. Why did I do that? I had planned all week that I would go and see Mum yesterday, but at the last minute I decided to take Lizzie to a new movie that had come out. It was a last minute decision that I was instantly regretting.

Mum was an epileptic and had been put into hospital three weeks earlier to get her medication changed. She needed to be in hospital to see if any adjustments to the medication were needed to keep the epilepsy controlled. It was while she was in hospital that she had fallen, broken her right hip and been put into the orthopaedic ward. She had an operation on her hip three days earlier and had been given a blood transfusion the night before she died of a pulmonary embolism.

Along with my sister Lesley and my brother Tony we helped and supported Dad around the time of the funeral and for a few days afterwards to help sort Mum's clothes and to make sure Dad would cope. Barry and I stayed for about a week after the funeral as we all came to grips with the reality that Mum was no longer with us.

For the next couple of months, we made regular trips back to Pahiatua to make sure that Dad was managing on his own. He had a nice group of friends from the RSA and he had played golf and bowls for years. Even though it was hard for him, he had friends around who helped him adjust to life without Mum.

Once we knew Dad was managing, we were able to ease off going over to Pahiatua every week and started enjoying life in Wanganui. I liked working at the maternity annexe and, after a year of working on the antenatal/postnatal ward, I started in the delivery suite.

It was a wonderful time of learning and consolidating my knowledge. I was becoming more confident in my ability as a midwife. Since the pace of work was reasonable, it was a time when I could learn with minimal stress and it was lovely to be able to spend time with the women I was caring for.

By the time I was rostered on to delivery suite, I was ready for more of a challenge and I looked forward to being with women in labour and supporting them when they gave birth to their precious babies.

Back Home

WE HAD BEEN LIVING IN Wanganui for nineteen months and our house back in Pahiatua had not sold, despite all our marketing efforts and prayers. We wanted to make Wanganui our new home but it was not to be. Taking a long look at our life, we felt that we could not move on and buy a house while ours was not sold, so we decided to go back to Pahiatua. Most would say that was a backward step and at the time we felt maybe it was, but we had little choice.

A lot had happened while we were in Wanganui. Dad had a heart attack soon after we arrived and then Mum died later that year leaving Dad alone. Our first grandchild, Petra, was born in 1995 at the end of our first year in Wanganui, and Angela had a baby girl named Meika in the following August. I missed my father and being able to call in and see him whenever I wanted. Now that he was on his own, it might be nice to be back where I could see him more often.

Elizabeth was nine years old and still missed her friends from Pahiatua terribly. She never wanted to move to Wanganui, so she was thrilled at the prospect of being home again and living in the house she never wanted to leave. She made a point of contacting all her friends and it was like a reunion when we arrived home. For me, it was like a defeat. I felt like I had failed because I hadn't been able to make a new life in a new town where we had a chance of a new beginning. Barry was ambivalent as to whether he stayed or returned to Pahiatua. It was me who had wanted to move so I could work in Wanganui as a new midwife.

I had grown so much as a midwife during my time in Wanganui. There was a wide range of experiences gained – from natural births to more complicated cases involving epidurals, assisted deliveries and caesarean sections. There were women who required closer monitoring, like those who had medical problems such as diabetes and high blood pressure, so I had gained a broad knowledge.

Again, the decision of where to work had to be made. I had always wanted to become an independent midwife when I felt ready. Now it seemed a perfect opportunity to take that step. Determined that moving back to our home town would not be a backward step, I became excited at the idea of setting up my own midwifery practice.

I couldn't wait to get back and start getting organised. Being an independent midwife was far more appealing than travelling to Palmerston North for work. The 40 minute journey each way while doing shift work held little appeal. While there were no criteria for becoming an independent midwife once registered, I felt that I had enough experience from working at Wanganui Hospital to do so.

Barry and I talked a lot about how it was all going to work. We decided that I would work from our home. The house was big enough. There was a second lounge by the front entrance with a bathroom across the passage that I could use as my consulting area – it was ideal. I could do my consulting at home, with privacy and minimal disturbance to the family. Plus, if there were any women who didn't keep their appointments, I could fill in time doing things around home.

Setting up practice was huge but exciting. The lounge was refurbished and new couches were purchased, along with curtains and cushions. I bought a cane basket and filled it with toys for the pregnant mothers' children to amuse themselves. The consulting room was cosy and inviting. I was sure the woman would love it. The bathroom was also renovated in time, with a new spa bath, vanity unit and toilet.

I was busy over the next few weeks buying equipment for the practice, setting up an account for hospital supplies, and communicating with the laboratory and ultrasound scanning providers. It took all my time and endless trips to Palmerston North to ensure everything was done before I commenced.

One of the bedrooms at home was made into an office where I could do all the paperwork. An office desk was bought, along with a new computer and fax machine. We put up a bookshelf to house all of the textbooks and resources I had on matters related to midwifery.

I needed to advertise my existence, so I put an ad in the local paper. From the advertisement, women would know that there was a midwife in the area providing maternity care. Even though independent midwifery had been around since 1990 and it was now 1996, there were still women who didn't know their options – especially in rural areas where general practitioners had done maternity care for decades. The concept of a midwife caring for women from early pregnancy to six weeks post-partum was still foreign to many.

I decided I would cover the area from Eketahuna to Woodville, including Pahiatua, and about an hour out to the coast east of Pahiatua. This included three towns and the surrounding farmland that included some smaller rural communities. Every household in Pahiatua and surrounding areas received the free local Bush Telegraph newspaper, so my advertisement would be seen. Women could choose to have their baby delivered at either Pahiatua Hospital or Palmerston North Hospital, and I offered homebirths for low-risk women.

In my naivety I never expected any opposition when I opened my midwifery practice. In fact, I had thought the opposite – that a midwifery service would be welcomed with open arms in the area. No doubt the women were pleased, but health professionals in town were less enthusiastic.

My interview for an access agreement to Pahiatua and Palmerston North Hospitals was intimidating to say the least. My confidence turned to nervousness and fear when I walked into the room to face a panel of 'judges'. The panel was comprised of four health professionals, including the midwifery manager of Palmerston North Hospital, the medical superintendent for maternity services, the manager of a small nearby hospital and a core midwife.

"What would you do if you had a baby born that needed resuscitating?"

"What would you do if you needed to transfer a woman in labour?"

"What would you do if a woman started having a post-partum haemorrhage?"

"What would you do if a woman ruptured her membranes and there was meconium-stained liquor?"

"In what circumstances would you consult an obstetrician?"

The questions kept coming relentlessly. It was as if I was sitting a verbal examination for state finals. I answered the questions knowing my ability to practice as an independent midwife hinged on this interview. When I left the room I was shaken, but confident I had answered their questions correctly. I didn't think there would be any problems until a few days later. I received a letter saying my application had been declined. No reason given. Initially, I was stunned. After considering how to respond for a few days, I wrote a letter appealing the decision. Fortunately, they reconsidered my application and I was granted an access agreement for both Pahiatua and Palmerston Hospital.

The hostility became more apparent when I visited Pahiatua Hospital to talk to the midwives there. As I walked in the back door and along the corridor, I heard the voice of a local general practitioner yelling in his Welsh accent.

"We don't want any independent midwives working in this town. You will close the hospital!"

I couldn't believe what I was hearing. I kept walking and didn't turn around. I made my way out the end door and walked back to my car without seeing anyone. I was stunned to think that setting up my midwifery practice could cause so much hostility. All I had wanted to do was provide a service for the women of the area. After all, this was my home town for goodness sake. What was the problem?

My mind flashed back to when Shelley died. The pain I had suffered started to resurface. Tears started to flow until it was torrential. I sat in the car mulling over what I'd just heard.

'No,' I thought. 'I won't give up. I won't give up my dream. I will do this for my daughter – my daughter who never had a chance at life. I wanted to be the best midwife I could possibly be and with God's help I would do it.'

After the tears subsided and I calmed down at home, a steely resolve replaced the tears. I would be the best midwife I could possibly be and give women the best care possible, no matter what opposition I might encounter. I knew now that it wouldn't be easy. There was opposition from people I never expected – but at least I knew my foe.

Early Days

BEING BACK IN PAHIATUA WAS nice in a lot of ways. It was nice to have Dad living just a block from us and to be able to call in when we were passing by. He enjoyed the impromptu visits and was managing well on his own. Dad started spending time with Kath a few months after Mum died. She was also living on her own after her husband died suddenly. Dad and Kath had known each other for years, but now that were on their own, they found companionship and friendship.

Every Saturday night they would get together and share a meal. It was lovely for Dad to have someone to share his life with. They continued to live in their own houses, but enjoyed going out together and spending time with each other. Having Kath in his life meant that Dad was not so reliant on us and we were pleased to see him happy again. He remained very social and active, playing golf and bowls, and spending time with his mates at the RSA.

Barry and I felt we needed a holiday before I started work. So we went with Lizzie and Dad to the Bay of Islands for two weeks. It was a part of New Zealand we had never been to before. We had a lovely time exploring the area and every day Dad would get the map out and look at what we were going to do that day. It was a lovely break before starting a new chapter in our lives.

When I arrived home and checked my messages on the phone, two women had rung wanting to book me as their midwife. My heart was encouraged that word was getting out. Golly, two women had rung to book me as their midwife. I couldn't wait to ring them back the next day and make appointments to see them and do my first bookings.

The local midwives at the Pahiatua Hospital were pleased that I would be doing low-risk deliveries there, with the threat of hospital closure looming. If I delivered a few more babies there, it might help ward off the inevitable. Unfortunately, nothing could stop the tide of change and the last baby was born at Pahiatua maternity annexe on June 20th 1998, just prior to the closure of the hospital on June 30th.

It was a privilege to guide Baby George into the world and have Sister Southgate beside me. Sister Southgate – now known to me as Gwenda – the midwife whom I had worked with all those years ago was now a lovely friend and colleague. The closure of the hospital was a sad time for all those who had worked there over the years. It was a fate experienced by many small hospitals throughout the country.

Since I was 40 minutes from a major hospital, I had to be prepared for any eventuality. When I set up practice, I gathered all the equipment I might need for unexpected events. In addition to the equipment I needed for antenatal and postnatal visits, I also had linen packs, birth packs, oxygen and resuscitation equipment with me at all times. I bought a large fishing tackle box with compartments that held all the supplies and drugs that might be needed for a birth.

I started meeting with midwives from Palmerston North and would regularly go over to the networking meetings that were held every fortnight. It was nice to have the connection with midwives in Palmerston North who could give support, encouragement and knowledge. It also meant that I wasn't so isolated.

The midwives were enthusiastic about meeting me and as I started attending the meetings regularly and building relationships with them, they started to refer women to me who lived in my area. Tungane, a homebirth midwife based in Dannevirke, started going to the meetings for the same reasons that I did. She had begun booking women for homebirths around the Dannevirke area and asked if I would back her up as a second midwife. I was happy to do so and pleased that we had a common goal of supporting women in the rural community.

Despite the opposition I had from some quarters, the phone started ringing and after a few months I had an adequate caseload. The numbers slowly built up from one or two a month to four to six a month. The advertising was working. As I started looking after more women, the care I gave became well known and more women started ringing and booking with me.

I saw women at the clinic I had set up at home from 9am until 3pm most days. The appointments were an hour long for the first visit and 30 minutes for a routine antenatal appointment, which gave me enough time to check the woman and baby and answer any questions the woman might have. If a woman missed an appointment for some reason I was able to do things that needed doing around home until the next appointment came.

Most of the postnatal visits I would do in the woman's home. Checking on the woman and how she was coping with a new baby, including breastfeeding and making sure the baby was gaining weight. I would travel out to her house, unless she lived very rurally and was coming into town anyway. Sometimes that would mean an hour's travel there, an hour for the visit and an hour home again.

It took time to adjust to being on call 24 hours a day, seven days a week. I had a cell phone and was always available, always within reach. As the first women I had booked approached their due dates, I found myself unable to sleep, wondering if the phone would ring any minute. I would fall asleep and then look at the clock to discover it had only been an hour since I last looked at it.

"What's up?" Barry would say when I would get up, put my dressing gown on and go and watch television for an hour or so hoping I would become tired enough to fall asleep. Gradually, though, I settled into a better sleep pattern and it didn't worry me so much that the phone could ring at any time. I got used to being on call and relaxed into it. Sometimes I would lie awake if a woman had rung me just as I was going to bed to say she was in early labour. I would toss and turn all night, waiting for her to ring back and say she needed me to go see her.

My life began to have more of a routine. It was only when I was called out after hours or when I had been up all night at a birth that I would have to rearrange my diary and appointments might have to be moved. Seeing women during school hours meant that I was home when Elizabeth came home from school, so it wasn't too disruptive, even though I was on call. It didn't take too long before it felt like we had never left Pahiatua and living in Wanganui became a distant memory.

The Family Down the Road

WITH ADVERTISING AND WORD OF mouth, news spread that there was an independent midwife in the community. There was a Maori family who lived down the road and had six girls. They had gone to the same nearby school as Angela. One day there was a knock on the door and, on opening it, I saw a tall, slender Maori girl standing there. I recognized her as one on the Rahui girls. She paused for a minute as she gathered her thoughts.

"Would you be able to look after me? I'm having a baby. It's due in October and Mum said you might be able to take me," she seemed a little nervous as she stood there waiting for my reply.

"Would you like to come in?" I said, trying to help her feel at ease.

"I'll just go and get my diary and have a look at my bookings," I said and went to the bedroom to grab my diary.

"What day are you due in October?" I asked.

"Well, I went to the doctor a couple of weeks ago and he ordered me a scan. I have had that and the scan said I was due on the 5th of October. He took some bloods as well and some swabs," she said, becoming more relaxed as she talked.

"That would be fine; I'd love to look after you." I said as I checked my diary.

"Do you want to make an appointment now for next week and we can do your booking then? I can get the scan report and all the blood and swab results for when you come for your booking visit. I can't remember, though – which one are you now?" I said, feeling I should know all the names of the girls but realising that they all looked very similar.

"I'm Patty, the second one in the family. My real name is Patricia, but they call me Patty for short. The eldest, Hine, has left home. She is living at Himitangi Beach, but the rest of us girls are still at home," she replied.

"Ok, Patty. We'll book the appointment for next Wednesday morning at ten o'clock if that suits and I'll get the results from the laboratory and scan result for then."

"Is it alright if I bring my mother, as she wants to come?" She stood up and prepared to go.

"It will be nice for your mother to come," I said.

Patty and her mother came for her appointment the following week and we went through her medical history and reviewed her results. I explained the maternity system and what services were offered. They took it all in and were thankful for all the pamphlets and information I gave them on keeping well during pregnancy.

"We should be able to hear the baby's heartbeat," I said after all the paperwork had been completed.

Both their eyes lit up when they heard the heartbeat sounding out from the doppler.

"Wow," Patty said. "It's fast."

"Well, they always sound fast," her Mum chipped in.

The pregnancy went well and Patty usually turned up for the

regular appointments. If she didn't show, I would call into the house as I was passing and let her mother know I needed her to come see me or ring in order to make another appointment.

It was late in September when Patty went into labour. The phone rang in the middle of the night. It was her mother.

"Patty's been in labour for a few hours now. I think it's about the time that you should come. She's contracting every four minutes and they're lasting about a minute."

"I'll be there shortly," I replied.

I quickly got dressed, gathered what I needed and drove the short distance to their house. The whole household was awake, either in the kitchen or with Patty in the bedroom. As I made my way past all the people, I wondered how they could all live comfortably in such a small house. It was the most basic of houses with only three bedrooms, but they seemed happy and managed with the confined space.

"You're well on the way," I said as I examined Patty. "You're already five centimetres and the contractions are well established. We might as well head off to the hospital."

Doreen, Patty's mother, said, "I wouldn't let her ring you too early. I wanted to make sure she was in proper labour before we rang you."

"No, you did well. You're such a great support for her since you've been through it many times yourself. You know what you're doing," I said, reassuring her.

I was impressed by the way Doreen supported Patty throughout the pregnancy and in labour. She had been through it before and knew what was normal. I thought back to when Doreen had her first two babies when I was working at Pahiatua Hospital as a nurse aide.

'That seems so long ago now,' I thought to myself.

We drove to Palmerston North Hospital with Patty, her mother and boyfriend in one car and me following close behind in mine. I always found this was the easiest way. If they needed to stop for any reason, I was right behind them.

When we got to hospital, Patty continued progressing well and had a baby daughter four hours later.

The little girl came out screaming and weighed 2,950 grams. Doreen couldn't wait to get her hands on her granddaughter. She rocked and cuddled her as I tended to Patty. The baby's father seemed happy to just take it all in and wasn't worried that Doreen got the first hold. I wondered if he would ever get a look in.

I knew that Doreen wanted the best for her children and grandchildren and I was sure that the baby was in good hands. She was the matriarch of the family. The whole family held her in high regard. Mum knew best and they would listen to her advice and what she had to say.

'What a straight-forward, normal birth,' I thought. 'Wouldn't it be great if they were all so easy?'

Patty wasted no time coming home. The next day I got a ring from the hospital letting me know she had gone home. I was pleased, since going half a block down the road to do postnatal visits was preferable to tripping over to Palmerston North Hospital each day.

Patty was the first Rahui girl that I looked after, but soon they were coming to me one by one. Some of the girls I looked after twice. I cared for one or more of the girls every year that I was practicing. When I visited Patty with her second baby two years later, the girls' father was on a bed in the lounge. He was dying of cancer and had been sent home to spend his last few weeks at home with his family.

Even though it was a sad time, I felt privileged to be part of their lives and that they appreciated the care I gave them as a family.

One night there was a loud knock at the door. I got Barry to go and answer it, not sure who was knocking so loudly on the front door in the middle of the night. There was a Maori man standing at the front door and a bicycle lying in the driveway.

"Could you please tell the midwife to come? My cousin is in labour around in Duke Street."

Barry took the address and the woman's name and came and told me what was happening.

"I don't know that name at all," I said. "She's not one of my women."

I got out of bed, got dressed and went to the address anyway and there in the house were members of the Rahui family. Their cousin had been visiting and gone into labour, so they had called me to tend to her.

Noeline was well established by the time I arrived and, since I didn't know anything about her, I called an ambulance to take her to the hospital. I went with her and she had the baby soon after we arrived. I talked to her about her history after the fact. She lived in a town two hours away and this was her third baby. Soon after the birth, Noeline and her partner moved to Pahiatua and I ended up being her midwife for three more of her children.

Over time, some of the Rahui daughters moved into their own places as they became more independent. They always got me to look after them and Doreen was always there when each grandchild was born. Some women have a tough time in labour, but not the Rahui girls. They all seemed able to deliver their babies with ease, or it might have been Doreen telling them to toughen up that did it.

As time went on, there were other families like the Rahuis who chose me as their midwife. I would care for all the family members, cousins and extended family. Sometimes I would be doing a postnatal visit and I'd be asked to see another family member who had just found out she was pregnant. They would embrace me and make me their family midwife. It was a privilege to be part of a family's most precious moments.

The Night Princess Diana Died

BARRY AND I DECIDED TO go to Wellington and see Kelvin and Veronica for the day. It was one of those spur of the moment decisions when we decided we wanted to visit family. We had not been to see Kelvin for a while and a quick trip down to Wellington for the day would be a nice interlude. It didn't seem that likely that someone would call, although one could never tell. The unexpected was always possible and I had to be prepared for any scenario. If a woman had booked with me, I was obligated to be available if there was any problem and she needed to be checked out. This could happen at any time during pregnancy – vaginal bleeding, decreased fetal movements or unexplained pain were just a few of the many possibilities.

I asked Linda to cover for me. She was happy for me to ring her if a woman rang me who needed to be checked out or may have come into labour. The arrangement seemed a lot easier than taking all my notes to Linda and, if I was needed, the drive was only two hours away.

Barry, Elizabeth and I enjoyed a nice day visiting Kelvin and Veronica. Their new baby, Shalom, was only a few weeks old. She was becoming so interesting, as her personality started to emerge. She was smiling all the time now and would make a squealing noise when she became excited or when you talked to her. They now had two beautiful daughters. Petra, their first daughter, was twenty months old and loved to see Nana and Pop.

We travelled back home in the early evening. I dozed in the passenger seat of the car with my eyes closed, but fully aware of the twists and turns in the road. Darkness had fallen and black was all that could be seen outside the car window. Barry had 'Elvis's Greatest Hits' playing in the background, as he often did when he was driving the car. He had always been a huge fan of Elvis and the songs brought back memories of another era and his younger days.

'It's Now or Never' had just started to play.

'It's now or never.
Come hold me tight.
Kiss me my darling.
Be mine tonight.
Tomorrow will be too late.
It's now or never.
My love won't wait.'

Through the sound of Elvis, I heard another sound in my dozing state, I suddenly realised that my phone was ringing. I turned Elvis down and pressed the answer button.

It was Veronica's voice on the phone.

"Princess Diana has died. It just came on TV."

"What! What happened?" I asked, stunned at what I was hearing.

"She died in a car crash in Paris just a short time ago. It was a special announcement. They don't know exactly what happened, just that she is dead and it was a car accident. I thought you would want to know."

"Oh no! I can't believe it. That's so tragic. Thanks for ringing. We'll turn on the television when we get home."

"Princess Diana has died." I turned to Barry.

For the rest of the journey home all I could think of was Princess Diana. That she had died so suddenly, so young and without warning. Silence filled the car as we made our way home. I couldn't stop thinking about the young sons she had left behind and the tragedy of her passing. She was such a beautiful, lovely person whose life had been unexpectedly cut short. I couldn't wait to get home and turn on the TV so I could see what had happened and how.

I kept thinking of the news I had just heard, going over in my mind how this could have happened. I was wide awake now, willing the car to go faster so I could be home and hear the news. When we got home, I rushed inside and turned on the television.

"Go and get yourself ready for bed," I instructed Elizabeth as we got inside.

I was camped in front of the news. The lounge light was on and the television on before Barry even came inside. There was a message flashing across the screen saying that Princess Diana had died and bits of news came on at regular intervals. The details were still sketchy. Princess Diana and her boyfriend Dodi Al-Fayed had been killed in a car accident in a Paris tunnel while trying to escape the paparazzi.

"I'll put the jug on," were Barry's first words as he came through the door.

We kept watching the broadcasts for at least an hour. I sat glued to the screen in front of us as we drank tea and ate some cake that I had in the tins. Updates were repeated at regular intervals, but no further information was known.

"I think I'll get to bed," Barry said as no more information seemed to be coming through.

"They'll know more in the morning, I'm sure. The news will be full of it for days and weeks to come," he said as he started to make moves to get out of his chair.

Satisfying myself that I'd not be missing any new information, I also conceded that there would be no more news until the morning and made my way to bed.

I lay in bed thinking about the lovely day we had spent with our beautiful granddaughters and how the news of Princess Diana's death had been like a bolt out of the blue – shocking everyone in the world. I would never forget those moments, when I heard the terrible news that would overshadow an otherwise perfect and idyllic day.

The sound of the phone ringing woke me from a deep sleep. I turned over and looked at the clock. The time said 10:32pm, so I can't have been asleep long. Tungane, the midwife from Dannevirke, was on the phone.

"Hi, Julie! I have Karen in labour. She's in the pool now and the contractions are coming strong. It would be good if you could come over now. It's her fourth baby so it might not be too long. I've been here for about three hours and everything is going well."

I had met Karen a few weeks ago after Tungane asked me to be her second midwife. If I was going to be the second midwife at a homebirth, I used to meet the woman around 36 weeks, so at least

I would have met the woman and know where she lived. It also gave the woman a chance to meet the other midwife who would be attending her birth.

"Ok, I'll be there as soon as I can," I said, jumping out of bed and throwing some clothes on.

Every night I laid my clothes out in case I was called, so I could dive out of bed and quickly get dressed. Rummaging around in the dead of night would have wasted time and possibly woken Barry, although nothing short of an atomic bomb would normally stir him.

A quick splash of water on my face, shoes on and I was out the door. Driving over to Dannevirke was becoming more familiar. I had decided not to obtain an access agreement to Dannevirke Hospital, but I was happy to support Tungane and be second midwife for her homebirths.

The map I had drawn with instructions on how to get to Karen's house was on the passenger's seat. I made sure I knew how to get to the house when I visited at 36 weeks. As I entered Dannevirke, I stopped the car and quickly checked that I knew how to get there. Funny, how easy it is to get disorientated and lose your way at night.

I had learnt that the hard way and took no chances, even if I thought I knew the way. It wasn't worth getting lost. I always had instructions and a map, especially to houses in the country or in areas I was unfamiliar with.

A few minutes later, I was pulling up Karen's drive. The lights outside were ablaze. Tungane and I always had the outside lights lit up when we had someone at home in labour, so that the place could be spotted from a long way off.

As I entered the house, I could hear the encouragement of Tungane's voice in the next room. The moist air from the pool and the warmth of the house touched me as I came in. I slowly made my way into the room, so as not to disturb the peaceful and calm atmosphere. Karen was in the birth pool, unaware that another person had come in the room. Andy, Karen's husband, and Tungane were crouching around the pool, quietly supporting the woman doing all the work.

Tungane looked up and acknowledged me as I entered the room, smiling at me and thanking me for being there. There was always a bond of thankfulness present when a second midwife arrived. It meant a lot to know that you had support and another pair of hands to assist bringing this baby into the world.

I looked around to find the doppler so we could listen to the baby's heartbeat. Taking it, I put the transducer under the water and onto Karen's lower abdomen. The reassurance of a steady heartbeat sounded out. I listened for a minute and then pressed the off button.

"Can you just check the water temperature for me, Julie? Tungane said. "It has been ok but I haven't checked it recently."

I went and got a thermometer out of Tungane's equipment box.

I put the thermometer into the water and waited for the beep.

"36.7," I said. Do you want me to boil the jug and top the pool up with some hot water?"

"With the last few contractions, there have been signs of second stage so it is a good time to do it. Karen has been feeling a lot of bowel pressure and the sounds she is making are promising," Tungane said.

I went into the kitchen and flicked the jug on and then came back into the room where everyone was.

"I'll check the equipment if you like." I made my way over to the corner where Tungane had set up all her birth equipment. I undid the birth pack, containing a large kidney dish, two metal clamps, a pair of scissors and a packet of large swabs. I opened a pair of sterile gloves and a plastic cord clamp and added them to the opened birth pack. I turned on the oxygen cylinder, making sure the tubing and mask were properly attached. The equipment was set up on a thick blanket not far from the birthing pool.

Towels and baby clothes were over a heater nearby. I looked at the baby clothes, then went and touched them to feel how warm they were.

'How inviting and warm for a newborn baby to get dressed into,' I thought as I felt the warm, soft towels and clothes.

Another contraction started. I kneeled and waited with anticipation. Karen was pushing now and I reached for the sieve as a bowel motion came out into the water.

I went into the kitchen, got the boiling water and carefully poured some into the pool. I took the temperature again a few minutes later and the reading was 37 degrees – the ideal temperature for the baby to be born into.

It was only fifteen minutes later when I looked down and saw the baby's head, covered in black hair, pushing through the perineum.

'The baby will be here any minute,' I thought to myself as I made my way around the pool to where the equipment was set up.

"You're doing well, Karen. Baby will be here with the next contraction. Just keep your bottom well down in the water." Tungane came around to the birth pack and put a pair of gloves on.

With the next contraction, the head was out. The baby's head was clearly visible sitting between its mother's legs in the warm water. Then another contraction and the body slid into the water. Tungane guided the baby in the water until its whole body was born, then brought the baby to the surface. As he broke the surface of the water, his eyes opened and, as he looked around, Tungane placed him on his mother's chest. Karen lay in the water with her arms around her beautiful newborn.

"He's perfect," she said, looking between his legs to check whether she had a son or daughter. Andy knelt beside them and I handed him the camera to see if he wanted to take some photos.

"Can you take some?" he said as he knelt beside his wife stroking her hair.

I took the camera and started clicking, capturing the most beautiful of wonders. The baby just lay on his mother's chest making the occasional cry, settling into his mother and the warm water.

His body was pink and he moved his little legs, kicking into his mother's stomach. Tungane came around to the baby and felt the umbilical cord for the heart rate. There was no need to rush this moment. Mother and baby were safe, well and in a warm place. I continued taking photos so this precious moment would be captured. There was some blood in the water but nothing indicated that the bleeding was excessive.

Before the water cooled too much, we helped Karen out of the pool with the baby still attached to the placenta via the umbilical cord. As Karen lifted her legs over the side of the pool, the placenta appeared at the entrance of her vagina. I grabbed a large kidney dish and encouraged her to push as the placenta plopped into the dish.

We wrapped towels around Karen and the baby to stop them

becoming too cold. The room was warm and the heater was on full, but it was still cooler than in the pool. We led Karen to an area that was set up with pillows and blankets. There was a sheet on the floor with a blue waterproof sheet on top.

"Do you want to cut the cord, Andy?" I asked as Karen lay on the floor.

Andy came over and I handed him the scissors.

"Here, cut between the two clamps," I said, as I secured the clamps and held the cord between the two.

I took the baby and dried him while Tungane looked to see if the perineum needed any sutures. I wrapped up the little bundle and gave him to Andy to hold while our attention turned to Karen.

"There is a tear that needs to be sutured, Karen. Sorry about this, but it really needs to be done," Tungane said as she checked the perineum with some gauze squares.

"I always have to be sutured, ever since I had an episiotomy with my first baby. It always tears down the same place."

"I can see that," Tungane replied.

I looked in the birth toolbox and took out the suture material and instruments needed. The birth pack hadn't been touched, so I placed the suture material there for the procedure. Andy held the baby while I held a torch and Tungane made the repair. It was unfortunate that Karen needed sutures considering how well the birth had gone, but a tear is often unavoidable, especially given that she had torn there previously.

Once the suturing was done, Karen put the baby skin-to-skin and started to breastfeed her son. Karen had been a successful breastfeeder with her other three children, feeding all of them for well over a year. There was no assistance needed as mother and baby knew what they were doing.

I went into the kitchen to make everyone a cup of tea and toast. Andy came out to show me where everything was in the kitchen.

"Here is some cake that Karen made yesterday. I think she must have known something, as she cleaned the whole house and did some baking."

"Well, that's lovely," I said as I prepared a tray with the tea and cake. We sat down and enjoyed the tea and cake while the baby had a good feed. We enjoyed the moment with the family and shared their special time.

The baby had a long breastfeed and, after he came off, Tungane started checking the baby over, weighing him and doing an initial head-to-toe check. While Tungane checked the baby, I checked Karen's blood pressure, temperature and pulse rate. I checked her vaginal blood loss and gave her fundus a rub to make sure it was well contracted.

Tungane had to stay with Karen for two hours following the birth of the placenta. Once most of the work was done and there didn't look to be any problems, I decided to go. I left 30 minutes before the two hours was up.

It was only as I was driving home that I realised I had forgotten to mention about Princess Diana dying. I had no idea if they knew or not.

It was a night and a birth that would always be etched in my memory.

'No matter what happens, or who dies, life continues and babies keep being born,' I thought.

A Baby in the Gorge

THERE WERE TWO ROUTES TO Palmerston North Hospital from Pahiatua, but since the hospital was closer to the Manawatu Gorge route, I always chose to travel that way. The road was windy, with cliffs on one side of the road and a sheer drop down to the Manawatu River on the other, but it was flat. It was very picturesque as you drove around all the bends. Across the river was a railway line and bush that covered the cliffs up the other side. Sometimes you would catch the sight of a train weaving around the cliffs, ducking through the tunnels on the other side of the river. In the early morning or at dusk, with the sun filtering through the cliffs, it was a sight to behold – although most of the time my mind was not on the scenery.

Whenever a woman went into labour and needed to get to Palmerston North Hospital, I would follow her and her birthing partner to the hospital in my car. Usually, I would have assessed the woman at home first and if she was in established labour, we would make our way in convoy through the gorge, which was a few kilometres on the other side of Woodville. Once through the gorge, it would only be another fifteen minutes before we would arrive in Palmerston North. The journey from Pahiatua was about 40 minutes in total. For a woman in labour, it was a very uncomfortable journey.

Diane rang me in the afternoon to say that she had been contracting irregularly all day. She said she would get back to me when labour became more established. Later in the afternoon, I decided to ring her and see how the labour was going, since I hadn't heard anything. I became a bit anxious when there was no reply at her house and I couldn't reach her by cellphone. Diane lived on a farm an hour east of Pahiatua, so I couldn't just pop around to see her. I wondered what to do if I couldn't get hold of her. There was not a lot I could do, but wait for her to contact me. It was 30 minutes later when the phone rang. I felt relieved to hear Diane on the other end.

"Hi, Julie. We've arrived at Kay's house. The pains are a lot stronger now and coming more frequently. I'm in the bath and it would be good if you could come now."

"Ok, I'll be there as soon as I can," I replied.

She sounded like she was in good labour, so I got in the car and drove to her mother-in-law's house. When I arrived at the house, Kay took me into the bathroom where Diane and Ian were. The labour was really cracking on and the bath may not have been such a good idea, since it seemed to have got the labour going even more. Diane breathed heavily as she got out of the bath for me to examine her.

On examination, the cervix had thinned out and the bulging forewaters could be felt in front of the baby's head, pushing through the dilating cervix.

"We had better get going. You're already seven centimetres," I said.

It was one of those times where I wondered, 'Is she going to have the baby soon, or do we still have time to get to the hospital?'

It was a difficult call at the best of times. If we had decided to stay, the baby may or may not have arrived soon and we weren't prepared for a homebirth – although I did have all the gear in the car. At least with the membranes intact, we might still have enough time to make it to the hospital.

We set off with Diane and Ian in their car and me following behind in mine. We travelled to Woodville and then made a left turn towards the gorge. I tried to follow as closely as possible, keeping my eyes fixed on their car ahead. The cars weaved around the ever-winding road. It was dark now and it took all my concentration to track their vehicle and not lose it in the constant stream of headlights coming towards me. As we neared the end of the gorge, I saw their indicator lights flash and the car slowed down and pulled over to the side of the road.

I got out of my car and went around to the front passenger side of the car in front.

"I want to push," cried out Diane. I could see she was trying with all her might to control what her body was trying to do. Their vehicle was a large four-wheel drive and I wondered for a minute how I was going to get up into the vehicle, let alone deliver a baby.

"Diane, you're going to have to get out and get into the back seat of my car. I think that is the best way. I have a rug in the back and I'll be able to get my gear from the boot."

Ian and I slowly helped her down and led her back to my car. I left the front passenger door open, so we had a bit of light from the small light inside the car.

'Not the most ideal of birth suites, but it's the best we've got,' I thought.

"Just stay with her for a minute, Ian. I'll get the gear from the boot."

With that, I quickly grabbed my toolbox and some gloves. I was putting them on when another contraction came.

"I can feel the baby," she called out. "It's coming. I can't stop it."

I looked down to see the baby emerging from her vagina. Her pants were around her knees.

With my gloves still only half on, I guided the baby onto the car blanket. As the little boy started to cry, everyone breathed a sigh of relief.

"Well, he wasn't going to wait for anyone, was he," I said.

We took a moment to take it all in before I went to get some linen from the boot. I brought back some towels to dry the baby and soak up some the blood and fluid that seemed to be everywhere.

"That's a first – I've never had a baby born in my car before," I said.

"I'm so sorry about the mess," Diane said. "I just couldn't help it."

"Don't worry. Sometimes babies come quickly and they're not going to wait until we're in the hospital. It's unavoidable at times. I think the bath really got things going. I knew you were in strong labour, but it's always difficult to tell how close the birth is," I said looking down at mother and baby.

"Usually, though, if a baby comes quickly, all is well. So that's one thing." I said trying to reassure her.

"What did I have?" Diane asked, trying to see in the dark.

"We have a son," Ian said.

The new arrival was lying in Diane's arms, happy and content. The crying had stopped and he was just snuggling into his mother.

"I think we'll call the ambulance and they can come out and get us. That would be the safest. I'll let them know what has happened." I got my cell phone and rang for the ambulance to come. I also rang the hospital to let them know that the baby had been born on the way. I'd rung them before leaving the house, so they were expecting us.

It was not long before the ambulance arrived. I helped Diane and the baby into the back. There was no bleeding, so I decided to leave the placenta alone until we got to the hospital.

When we got to hospital, the placenta came out with a push from Diane as we were transferring her onto a bed in the postnatal ward.

Ian started ringing everyone to tell them what had happened and that all was well. While he was on the phone, I checked baby and mother.

"You don't have any tears, Diane," I said, checking the perineum to see if suturing was needed. The warm bath would have helped with stretching the perineum.

After getting Diane and Ian a cup of tea and some toast, I left them to bond with their new son. Diane had already put the baby on the breast.

I went to start the paperwork. Hospital notes needed to be written, as well as my own notes. The written notes on the pregnancy, labour and birth had to be recorded on the hospital computer programme, and the birth of the baby had to be registered. The paperwork was always time consuming. In addition to the notes that were written about the labour, which had to be meticulously accurate, there were notes recording the baby's details at the time of birth and the health and condition of the mother and baby.

We were required to stay with the woman and baby two hours following a birth, but it always took that long just to complete all the paperwork and fulfill all the legal requirements.

Diane and the baby stayed a couple of nights in hospital, since they lived so far out in the country. It was better to be well rested and have the breastfeeding going well before they headed home.

I enjoyed my time travelling out to Diane and Ian's farm to do the postnatal visits and there was some sadness when I finally discharged Diane and baby at six weeks.

Diane was not the only woman who had a baby born on the way to Palmerston North Hospital. Over the years, I had deliveries at various points on route. Fortunately, the baby came out screaming and in good condition every time. It was a question of timing and sometimes we just didn't have the time to get there. It was one of the challenges of working rurally and being 40 minutes away from the hospital. No matter how much planning we did, the baby had the last say as to when it would enter this world.

Breech Birth at Home

Rose had booked with me when she was eight weeks pregnant. It was her third baby and the previous births had gone well with no complications. The other babies had been born at a hospital in the Bay of Plenty. Rose, her partner and their children had moved into the area about four months ago and lived on a dairy farm about eight kilometres out of town. They were share milkers and had arrived at the start of the milking season. Rose was happy to come to my clinic at home for all her antenatal visits, since she lived out of town.

At each antenatal check, both mother and unborn baby were in good condition. The polycose test was high at 28 weeks, but a glucose tolerance test ruled out gestational diabetes. We talked about her birth plan during the visits. Rose wanted to deliver at Palmerston North Hospital, so I had booked her in for the birth there.

We talked about what would happen when she went into labour. I would come to her house and assess her and then we would travel to the hospital.

When Rose came for her weekly check at 38 weeks, she staggered up the stairs to my front door and seemed to be in a lot of pain when I opened it.

"What is wrong, Rose?" I said as I led her into the lounge area.

"I'm just so sore down there. I can hardly walk. The baby seems to be so low. I have to walk with my legs apart and I've got shooting pain down my legs."

I sat her down on the couch and she told me that it had been like this for a few days.

"How is it when you are sitting or lying down?" I asked.

"It's not so bad when I'm off my feet, but as soon as I stand up to walk I have pain in my pelvis and shooting pain down my legs," she replied.

Rose seemed more relaxed now as she sat on the couch chatting to me.

I went and got the 'smiley belt' that I had bought from a physiotherapist and asked her to stand as I put it around her back and secured it under her abdomen.

"Try this. It supports the weight of your baby and takes the pressure off your pelvis. Hopefully it should work for you. Also, try and rest as much as possible. The head must be very low."

"Thanks. I hope it works. It sometimes feels like the baby is just going to fall out." Rose sat back down on the couch.

"Can you lie down for me? I'll check the position of baby and its heartbeat," I said.

I started to palpate Rose's heavily-pregnant tummy. The head was so low that I couldn't feel it above the pelvis. As I moved my hands up to feel the top of her abdomen, I felt what might have been the head just under her ribs. I spent some time palpating her to determine if it was a head I was feeling or just a hard bottom, as sometimes it was.

I wasn't sure so I decided to get an ultrasound scan done to check the baby's presentation. I rang to make an appointment for as soon as possible. Since it was Friday, there was no appointment available until Monday morning.

"We will just have to go with that," I said to Rose. "Take this form and they will see you on Monday morning at 10:30am. I'm unsure how the baby is presenting and it could be in a breech position, so we will check and go from there. They will ring me with the result as soon as they have it and we can consult with a specialist if the baby is breech. In the meantime, rest as much as you can and keep the smiley belt on for support."

After the appointment finished, I showed Rose to the door. She was walking a lot better with the smiley belt in place and looked a lot more comfortable.

The following day was Saturday and my usual clean of the house. I spent the morning changing sheets, doing laundry, dusting and vacuuming. I always felt good after the big Saturday house clean. It was late in the afternoon when the phone rang.

It was Rose on the phone. "I have broken my waters. I was just getting up off the couch when I felt a gush of fluid go down my leg. I have put a pad on and there is still fluid coming out."

"Is the fluid clear, Rose?'

"Yes, it's clear and there was lots of fluid. There is no doubt my waters have gone."

"Has the baby been moving ok today? Have you had any contractions?" I asked.

"The baby is moving ok and I have had a few pains since my waters broke. I think I am definitely contracting. They are not that bad yet, though," Rose said.

I continued asking questions for a few more minutes. Rose seemed to calm and the contractions weren't coming too strong.

"Ok, Rose. I'll come out to see you and then we'll go to the hospital. We need to go together and it's better if I come to you first. We need to get over as soon as we can in case the baby is breech."

I quickly got a few things together and put it all in the car. I had to be prepared, since sometimes I would leave home and not return for hours. I always had a change of clothes, some toiletries and some snack food. I had been caught out before. I couldn't just pop home for a shower and something to eat, so I would be stuck otherwise.

I drove the eight kilometres to Rose's house and was met at the door by Bruce, Rose's partner.

"Rose is contracting very strongly now and has been since she called you. She is in the bedroom."

I went in and Rose was standing by the bed. She looked breathless and tired.

"The contractions started soon after my waters broke and they have gotten stronger and stronger. They are about three minutes apart now and lasting a while, taking my breath away."

Rose looked as if she had been breathing hard. Her face was flushed and she looked anxious.

"The movements of the baby have been ok, haven't they?" I asked.

"Yes, they have been fine. The baby has been pushing up under my ribs terribly since yesterday."

"I'll have to do a vaginal examination. I should be able to feel the presentation. It is a shame you were unable to have the scan yesterday. Can you lie on the bed for me?"

With that, another contraction came. Rose leaned over the bed and breathed intensely, concentrating as the contraction became stronger and stronger. Her face was red and sweat dotted her forehead.

"They are becoming so strong now. I want something. Can I have pain relief?"

"Lie on the bed when you can and I will do an examination and see where you're at. The contractions seem very intense already. You look to be in good labour."

I washed my hands and put some gloves on. Rose lay down on the bed, ankles together and legs apart.

"That's good, Rose. I'll be as gentle and as quick as I can."

I slowly put two fingers in her vagina and immediately found the cervix. I gently moved my fingers around the cervix. There was no mistaking the soft bottom pushing through the already four-centimetre dilated cervix. The flesh around the rim of the cervix was paper thin and the baby's bottom was so low that my fingers had hardly entered the vagina when they hit it.

Yes, Rose was in established labour and progressing fast. I pulled my fingers out and took the gloves off. Rose quickly got off the bed as another contraction came on.

I stood thinking about what to do. My heart was beating. A breech presentation and there was no way could she be driven to the hospital in convoy like we had planned. My mind was racing as I tried to consider all our options. I couldn't take her in my car with me driving, as I wouldn't be free to deliver the baby. Her partner couldn't even drive with the two of us in the back, as there is no way I could safely birth the baby in the car. It was just too risky because it was breech.

"Rose, you are dilating really fast and the baby is breech. I'm going to ring the consultant on call at Palmerston North Hospital and let him know what is happening. He will be on stand-by if we make it there before the baby is born."

I rang the hospital and it seemed like an age before the operator answered. Then it seemed like another age before I was put through to the obstetrician on call. I explained the situation – that I was over 40 minutes away, had a woman who was contracting strongly in established labour and that the presentation was breech.

"I'm about to call the ambulance but I wanted to let you know what was happening, so the team could be on standby for when we arrive."

"Put her in knee-chest position. That might slow her down a bit until the ambulance gets there."

"Alright, thanks."

I got off the phone and could hear Rose panting in the other room. I quickly went into the bedroom and asked her to kneel on the bed, put her head down on the bed and put her bottom in the air while I rang the ambulance.

I stepped out to ring 111. "Ambulance, police or fire?"

"Ambulance, please. Could I have an ambulance?"

"I have a woman here in strong labour with a breech presentation. We need an ambulance immediately to take her to Palmerston North Hospital. I'll hand the phone to her partner for directions on how to get here," I handed Bruce the phone.

"It's better that you tell them where to come, since you know the roads better. We can't have them getting lost."

My heart was still pounding and I could almost feel the adrenaline racing around my body. My mind was in a whirl as I started to think back to my emergency training on delivering a vaginal breech. It was something that was rare, since all breech presentations were delivered by caesarean section these days. My mind went back to Angela's birth, which was also a rapid labour and a vaginal breech.

Rose was on the bed, her bottom high in the air. 'It might give us some time,' I thought, 'but this baby seems to want out.'

I went over to Rose side and got the doppler to listen to the heartbeat.

"Baby has a strong heartbeat. Around 140 beats a minute. I have got the ambulance coming, Rose. Hopefully they won't be too long. Just stay in this position for now if you can. It might slow the labour."

Another contraction came. "I want pain relief, I want pain relief," Rose yelled at the height of the contraction.

All I could do now was wait for the ambulance and support Rose until it arrived. The baby's heartbeat was good and that was reassuring. I started to calm down a bit, knowing there was little I could do. I prayed silently.

The contractions kept coming intensely and the knee-chest position seemed to be having little effect. I kept listening to the baby's heartbeat at regular intervals.

There was calmness in the room – everything that could be done was done and it was out of our control. Rose responded to my back rubs and started coping better with each contraction. Bruce got some ice cold water for Rose to drink and a cold flannel for her forehead. Rose withdrew inside herself more and rested between the contractions. The panic was gone. With each contraction, Rose's breaths became more laboured as the intensity grew.

Thirty minutes later, just as I heard the ambulance back into the driveway, Rose started grunting as a contraction eased off. The telltale signs of second stage had begun. Two ambulance officers knocked at the door and were let in by Bruce.

Ngaire and John came in and I went to greet them.

"I think we are in second stage now. I'll just check her and see." I was relieved to see some familiar faces. Just having them there with me helped.

"You are fully dilated now, Rose. I think it would be best if you came on the floor and leaned over this chair." There was no point trying to slow things down now. The baby would have to be born at home.

Rose kneeled on the floor and leaned over a chair as I had asked her to. With the next few contractions, she pushed and it wasn't long before the buttocks became visible through the perineum. Meconium was coming out as the buttocks were being squeezed. I put the linen and birth pack on the floor beside me. Ngaire and John came in and stood by the bed.

"What do you need, Julie?" John asked.

"I have oxygen and resuscitation equipment here – but have you got any nitrous oxide? She has been asking for pain relief and it might help her."

"Do you want some gas, Rose? They have it in the ambulance. You just can't use too much at this stage."

"Yes . . . Yes . . ." Rose replied.

John went and got the nitrous oxide cylinder out of the ambulance and handed the tube with the mouthpiece on the end to Rose.

Rose breathed on the gas for a couple of breaths and then pushed the baby down with each contraction. With each push, more of the baby's body edged its way out. Rose was kneeling upright, so gravity helped as Rose pushed. Rose was so controlled and the room was hushed. Only the sound of Rose pushing out her baby broke the silence.

Having Ngaire and John present certainly gave me a sense of security and reassurance. They stood at the ready for any request I had and watched in awe as the little bottom, then the legs and then the body slowly made its way out. No manoeuvres were required, just gravity and guidance with minimal assistance. The body was now dangling down as far as it could come with the head still inside.

'This is the tricky bit,' I thought. I instinctively put my hands inside Rose and placed them around the head of the baby to support it. With the next contraction, my hands gradually flexed and guided the head out – the baby was born.

There was a sigh of relief in the room as the baby was brought down to a towel and started to cry.

"Well done, Rose. You have a little girl and she looks perfect."

The sense of relief was overwhelming as I heard the baby cry and cry. Everyone in the room rejoiced and started talking about how lovely the baby was. The placenta was soon delivered and Rose put her daughter on the breast.

"Do you want to go to the hospital, Rose? We can go in the ambulance. Or do you want to stay at home?" I asked.

"I might as well stay here. Not much point going now," she laughed.

The ambulance crew left and I rang the hospital to let them know that the baby had been born and all was well.

"You were so wonderful, Rose. Well done. What a great achievement. You had a breech birth at home. Of course, I wouldn't recommend it next time, or to any of your friends, mind you."

I spent the next couple of hours checking baby and making sure Rose was well enough for me to leave. Blood loss and observations were all normal.

"I'll see you tomorrow. I'm sure I'll sleep well tonight. Ring me if there are any problems or if you need me beforehand."

I left the house singing in my heart, so thrilled that all had gone well and thankful for a wonderful outcome.

Baby Born in Bedroom

TRACEY RANG ME AT EIGHTEEN weeks to let me know she was pregnant again and wanted to book me as her midwife. This was the second time I had cared for Tracey and the first birth had gone well. She was only in labour for six hours and the birth had been very straightforward. When she went into labour, Tracey and her husband came to my house and we travelled to the hospital together. When we arrived, she was already seven centimetres dilated and in very strong labour. After only an hour and 45 minutes at the hospital, she gave birth to a healthy baby boy weighing 3,600 grams. He was a vigorous baby and cried lustily at birth. What a joyous sound that was – the cry of a newborn baby. I couldn't think of a more lovely sound in the world. For a midwife attending the birth, it was precious music to the ears. Everyone would always relax after the baby let out those first lusty cries to let everyone know they were alive and well.

It was an announcement to the world saying, "I'm here, I've arrived".

Since Tracey lived way out in the country, approximately an hour's drive from Pahiatua, she decided to stay in hospital for a couple of days to make sure that the breastfeeding was going well. Mother and baby were well and breastfeeding was becoming established when Tracey was discharged home on the third day.

The following day, I journeyed to the homestead where they lived. It was a relaxing hour's drive from Pahiatua on narrow roads, mostly sealed but sometimes on gravel, through gorges, over bridges and around the hilly countryside dotted with flocks of sheep and herds of cows. Every few kilometres, there would be a homestead, proving that there was life out here in the middle of nowhere. The countryside was beautiful and green. Sometimes I would pass through communities that contained only a pub, a church and maybe a hall, then scattered houses for another few kilometres.

50 years ago when transport was not so easy and people were content to stay close to where they lived, these were thriving communities. Now, though, life was different. Regular trips to town and to the city replaced the times of self-sufficiency and the country store.

After a few turns up roads that were off the beaten track, I arrived at a gate with the number 520 written on a fence post in bold, red lettering.

'Yes, this is it,' I thought stopping to check my scribbled instructions of the roads to follow and how to get there. I turned up the long driveway that led to Tracey and Rob's home. The driveway wove another kilometre over unsealed dirt road until at last the house was in sight. The vision of the house broke through the trees. The ground that had been rough and stony became smooth and the farmland on either side of the driveway became rolling lawn up to the house in the distance. A tennis court in a state of disrepair was to the right at the edge of the rolling lawn.

The driveway led me to the front doorway of the large, old homestead that must have been built nearly 100 years earlier. I walked up the wooden steps to the large doorway that opened onto a veranda. There was a swinging seat that would have seated three, which looked out to the driveway and a view of the countryside beyond. Rhododendron trees of every shape and colour lined the edge of the lawn and the gardens. My surroundings spoke of old money, of prosperity and glamour, of a time gone by. Tracey and Rob were the third generation to have lived on and tended this very land, dedicating their lives to farming, isolation, long trips to town and a car that was permanently dirty from the gravel roads. They had to get in the car just to see their neighbours a few kilometres down the road. It was an hour's travel to Pahiatua and the nearest city was another 40 minutes on top of that.

I knocked on the door and was warmly invited in by Tracey. A hot cup of tea and cake were offered. How could I refuse such warm country hospitality? We chatted as I checked on Mum and baby. I asked all the necessary questions to ensure that all was going well. It was an hour visit covering all things related to their health. It was nice to recharge before the hour long drive back home again.

I visited a couple of times in the first week and then weekly until mother and baby were discharged at six weeks. Both Tracey and Baby James were doing well and breastfeeding was well established. I imagined this little boy being brought up on the farm. As soon as he could walk, he would be riding on the quad bike checking on the sheep on the rolling green countryside with his Dad.

I was delighted when Tracey rang me to care for her a second time. Since Rob and Tracey made regular trips to town, they were happy to come to the house for the antenatal visits. All the blood tests, swabs and routine antenatal checks could be done from the clinic at home. I would take the samples and request form to the medical centre, where the courier would pick them up each day to take to the laboratory in Palmerston North. It was only the ultrasound scans that would have to be done at Palmerston North. It was a perfect arrangement for both of us. It would only be when Tracey went home after the birth that I would travel out to her place as I did with her first baby eighteen months earlier.

Antenatally all went well. Apart for a repeat scan at 34 weeks to check a low-lying placenta, everything was on track for a normal birth. The scan came back showing that the placenta had conveniently moved up. Tracey was healthy throughout her pregnancy. When we discussed her birth plan at 36 weeks, we decided that when Tracey went into labour she would come to my house and we would travel to the hospital together, as we had with the first birth.

I was woken from a deep sleep when Tracey rang me one night at 2:45am.

"Hi, Julie. I have just had a large, bloody show and have been contracting regularly, so we have decided to leave now. We will see you at your place in about an hour. Is that ok?"

"Alright, I will see you soon." With that, I hung up the phone and went and had a shower. It seemed a long time to be waiting in the middle of the night. I went into the kitchen and made a cup of coffee. I began thinking about all that I might need and went through a checklist in my mind.

'Yes, I had filled the car up yesterday and Barry had checked the oil and water on the weekend. Yes, I had a sterilised birth pack, oxygen and linen bundle in the car. The large toolbox with all my homebirth equipment was in the boot, as well as my antenatal and postnatal bags.'

An hour had passed since Tracey had first rung when the phone once again disturbed the quiet of the night.

"Julie, the contractions are really strong and I want to push. I haven't been able to ring because there has been no cell phone coverage."

"Where are you now?" I asked.

"We are just coming into town on Tiraumea Road." The panic in Tracey's voice was palpable.

"Ok, come right up to our back door and I'll meet you there. Drive around the back."

I quickly hung up and went into the spare bedroom that was off the main lounge and started pulling the top covers off the bed. I ran outside and brought the birth gear and linen pack in from the car. I pulled out a waterproof sheet and covered it with a draw sheet then placed them over the bottom sheet of the bed. I ripped open the birth pack and put it at the end of the bed, turned on the oxygen, tested the ambubag and put the toolbox with all my homebirth provisions on the floor.

I ran down to the bedroom and started shaking Barry to wake up.

"Wake up, someone is coming in strong labour and it sounds like she will birth here. Quickly, get dressed in case I need you."

I ran back to the kitchen and, as I opened the back door, a large Range Rover pulled up. Tracey got out as soon as the vehicle stopped. Stopping for a contraction, she breathed loudly and was unable to move.

"When this contraction goes, come up the steps and into the house. I have a bed ready for you."

"Ok, I want to push and have been holding on just to get here."

"It will be alright. You're here now," I said as I led her up the steps, through the kitchen and into the spare bedroom.

Tracey got on her hands and knees and lent over the back of the bed. I could see anal pouting and the perineum opening. With the next contraction, the head was visible and, with the next contraction, the head was born.

"You are doing great, Tracey. The head is out now. Are you ok?"

"Yes, ok."

"Slowly does it. Now just a gentle push and pant. Baby is coming."

I guided the baby out and placed her on a sheet. She took a breath and cried.

"You have a girl, Tracey. You have a beautiful baby girl."

Tracey turned around to meet her baby as we waited for the placenta to be born. I dried the baby and lifted her onto Tracey's chest.

"Thank you so much. We made it here. I was so scared we would have the baby before we got here."

I turned around to see Rob beaming from ear to ear.

"I drove as fast as I could, but it's not easy in the dark on the winding country roads." He said recounting the trip.

"No, you don't want to risk having an accident that's for sure." I said.

The time of the birth was 4:02am and they had arrived at the house at 3:55am. Tracey had first rung me at 2:45am.

The placenta plopped out eight minutes later and Rob cut the cord. Zara, as she was called quickly, latched onto the breast and started sucking. Tracey lay back, enjoying the moment, relieved it was all over. Barry went into the kitchen and made a cup of coffee for Rob while I wrote up the notes and mother and baby had their special time.

Zara weighed 3,520 grams when she had finished feeding and I was able to weigh her and check her out.

"You have a lovely, healthy daughter," I said, wrapping baby up. I gave her to Dad as I checked on Tracey.

The blood loss was settled and the fundus was well contracted.

"I just need to check if you need stitches, Tracey. Then you can go and have a shower."

I got a torch to have a look at the perineum.

"There is a tear that needs stitches. It has gone into the muscle layer and really should be sutured, but it's not a difficult repair. It shouldn't take too long to do."

Rob held the torch and assisted as I did the repair.

When the suturing was done, Tracey got up for a shower and, when she was dressed, came out into the warm lounge for breakfast.

"I feel like a new woman," she said as she sat on the couch by Rob and baby Zara.

The hallway door opened into the lounge and a very sleepy looking Elizabeth appeared at the door.

"Come and meet a brand new baby, Lizzie. She was born two hours ago in the spare bedroom."

Liz came over and gazed in wonder, looking bewildered at all the strange people in our house.

"Do you want some breakfast, Lizzie?"

"No, not yet. I'll wait a bit," was the reply.

Tracey, Rob and little Zara left soon after breakfast to travel home. As Tracey said, there was little point going to hospital now since all was well.

I drove out to their place the following day and visited regularly over the next six weeks. Tracey and Zara continued doing well and I felt a bit sad when my visits out to the country came to an end. Even though it was three hours in total to do a postnatal visit, there was something special about visiting a couple you had formed a bond with over the months that you cared for them. Apart from meeting them up town, you often never saw a woman again once they were discharged, unless they had another baby. I pondered the closeness and the intimacy of the time spent caring for a family. Sometimes you would know the most intimate details of their personal life, only to have the relationship end after the care was finished and your job was done.

Time Out

ANGELA WAS HAVING HER SECOND baby and I needed to be with her as the due date approached. My midwifery practice would have to come second in this instance. I was on call 24/7 unless I planned to have some time off, which had to be organised months in advance. Annie, a midwife whom I had worked with, helped me out numerous times when I needed to get away. She also supported me when I had homebirths and was faithful in being there for me. Even when I had called her too early for homebirths at times, she would always come without complaint.

I took two weeks off around the time that Angela's baby was due and Annie covered for me over that time. Angela was married to Kevin and they lived on a farm in a small Taranaki community called Okato, a three hour drive from Palmerston North. I arrived at Angela's prior to her due date and waited for the new addition to arrive. He, however, was in no hurry to meet us and was ten days past his due date when he decided to make his entrance.

Angela had an unplanned waterbirth at Taranaki Base Hospital. She had got into the birthpool for pain relief and was unable to move once in the pool. The warm water helped with the pain and she was able to relax. She stayed in the pool until second stage and then, finding it difficult to get out, stayed in the pool for the birth.

Because I was at Angela's before she was due, I had little time with Angela after Max was born. My allocated two weeks were nearly over and I had to get home to my practice. I stayed for as long as I could and Angela was home and settled in with the baby before I left. I felt a twinge of guilt and sadness as the time to go approached. Angela was managing well and breastfeeding was becoming established with little or no input from me, but I still felt a longing to stay and help out. How great would it be to just do as I pleased?

There was no choice, though, and Angela understood the commitment I had to the women I was caring for. Also, Annie had her own practice to care for, without the added burden of another caseload.

I returned home to Barry and Elizabeth. They had kept the home running in my absence and when I walked through the door everything was tidy and in order. They coped well and managed all the household chores with ease. They had driven over to Taranaki to see Max when he was born but, apart from that, they had been at home working and going to school.

"I'm so pleased that you're home," Barry said as I walked in the door.

"There have been a few women who have rung to book with you. I've put the phone numbers on your desk. I said when you'd be back and they seemed to be happy to wait until then. Also, others rang just to enquire about different things, so I gave them Annie's number. It has been quiet here otherwise. Lizzie and I went to the movies the other night. It was one that just came out. We really enjoyed it. Shame you couldn't come with us."

"Yes, well you know what happened when I went to the movies last time. I was called out as a woman went into labour," I said, remembering the reality of being on call 24 hours.

"That's right. Well you just have to take the chance or you wouldn't be able to do anything. Like when we had that dinner party when Debbie stayed. You were called out, but at least we made an effort. If you thought about being on call too much, you would do nothing and go nowhere." Barry said, reminding me of a couple of months before when I had a midwifery student staying from England for three weeks. We had dinner with a few friends and were eating the main course when we both had to leave to attend a woman in labour. In fact, there were two births that night. We had just finished being with a woman in Palmerston North Hospital when we had to attend a homebirth in Woodville.

The woman in Woodville rang just as a decision had been made that the woman in Palmerston North needed a caesarean section. I had to leave the first woman in the care of the hospital team, once I had prepared her for theatre, to attend the homebirth. Not an ideal situation. Normally, I would have stayed and gone to the caesarean section. This time, though, it was unavoidable.

At times juggling these unforeseen events was stressful. I wanted so much to be there for each woman, but there were times when someone would be let down.

I had no regrets, though, about putting my family first for important events like the birth of a grandchild. The break had recharged my batteries and it was nice to be home.

The following day I had a full clinic from 9am until 3pm. As soon as I had unpacked my suitcase, I rang Annie to see if I could come and pick up my notes. Annie lived in Palmerston North and I enjoyed the drive over as my mind went into rest mode. I knew the road well. Every corner, bend and hill was familiar.

Annie heard me pull up in the car and came out to greet me as I opened the door to get out.

"Come in for a coffee if you have time," she called out.

Annie and I had grown close over the years. I had mentored her when she was a student, followed her progress through her midwifery training and now she was an independent midwife herself. All the women loved her. She was always fully booked and would often have to turn women away. It was lovely to have her support.

"How was your break and how are Angela and the new baby?" Annie asked.

I filled her in on my time away, recounting Max's birth and the time I had with Angela and Kevin. We chatted and caught up with each other's news. Things were always happening in the midwifery community, so it was nice to hear what had been going on. Then she went and got my case notes. One by one, she went through the notes of the women she'd looked after while I was away, updating me if there were any problems.

She had delivered one of my women who had come into labour three weeks early, who unfortunately ended up having a caesarean section. I was disappointed I hadn't been there for her, but she still needed postnatal visits so I would see her soon.

"Well, you can't predict everything," I said. "Who would have believed that she would go into labour three weeks early?"

"She understands," Annie said. "She knows that it's unusual to go into labour so early."

The birth had not been an easy one. The woman had progressed really well and became fully dilated quickly but in second stage the baby didn't descend. It was an ordeal for all involved. The woman had an epidural and a syntocinon infusion to try and push the baby down, but it was to no avail. After many hours of labour and medical intervention to help the baby come out vaginally, it was stuck in the pelvis and would not budge, so an emergency caesarian section was called.

I was grateful to Annie for being there for the woman. I didn't want Annie to have such a tricky case to deal with in my absence. I tried to book time off when there was no-one due, but birth was never predictable.

I left with all my notes, knowing I would have to sort them for the morning clinic when I got home. I was tired and looked forward to a good sleep. I prayed that I wouldn't be disturbed in the night. Not tonight anyway.

When I got home, I saw the pile of mail stacked up for me to deal with. Barry had put all the midwifery mail in its own pile for me to sort when I returned. Apart from checking on blood and ultrasound results, the rest would have to wait until tomorrow after clinic. I needed to go to bed and crash.

The Journey Continues

I ROSE EARLY THE NEXT morning to get a head start. I had a full clinic, plus catching up on all the washing and chores as time permitted. Lizzie was used to organising herself and didn't need any help to get off to school. She had grown very independent, or maybe she just had to with her mother always either studying or working. It didn't seem to have affected her in a negative way, though, and she coped well. Even with her albinism and poor eyesight, she had done well at school and we were pleased with her progress.

Since I had been working as a midwife, we only had Elizabeth at home, which had made it easier to juggle work and family. Angela had been at secondary school when I was studying, but had left home before we went to Wanganui.

Looking back, I concluded that, if I had waited until Lizzie was older to do my training, I might have missed the opportunity entirely. I don't know what I would have ended up doing otherwise. I had no regrets and Barry had reinforced to me many times that he had no regrets either. He was really pleased I had gone and pursued my dream.

Our relationship had gotten better over the years. All the past hurts and troubles had long gone and we had both moved on. We had let go and let each other do our own thing, which seemed to have worked. It was weighted my way, though, as I seemed to want to do more than Barry. His personality was different from mine, so I suppose in that way we complemented each other. He was so stable and reliable. He kept the home going and was there whenever he was needed, especially for Elizabeth.

It worked well for the seven years that I practiced as an independent midwife. I was not sure how long I would continue. Sometimes I thought that I would like to be free and not be tied to my pager or phone. I constantly needed to be available for the women I was caring for. But it had been a very rewarding and satisfying time. I had loved being autonomous and having my own practice.

For a few months I pondered the future and how long I would continue. Over the past year, there had been a few stressful births that hadn't been pleasant. I had two women go into labour at the same time and I had to call in back up to assist me because they birthed within minutes of each other. I also had a newborn that needed resuscitating at a homebirth due to meconium aspiration, which was very stressful. The delivery had been very quick and my back-up midwife arrived fifteen minutes after the birth, so I had to manage on my own until she arrived. A few more grey hairs had grown that night.

Nothing was avoidable or predictable. It was just the way birth went sometimes. You had to deal with whatever came along the best you could at the time.

I got all my notes sorted for the women who would come to the clinic that day. It would be busy, especially since I had been away for a couple of weeks. I had three full days of clinic that week, leaving the other two days for home visits. I hoped no one came into labour during the daytime this week, as it would be tricky juggling the appointments.

"Are you ready for a busy day then?" Barry asked as I came out into the kitchen to get my breakfast and coffee.

"Yes, all good," I said. "It's was nice to see Angela and spend time with her, but I'm pleased to be back home."

"Are you ok, Lizzie? What have you got on today?" I asked.

"Just the usual classes, nothing that exciting," was the reply.

Elizabeth was at secondary school now. She had two more years left after this one, so it wouldn't be too long before she too would be leaving the nest. Lizzie had been like an only child in many ways and had enjoyed the benefits of being the only one at home.

"I should be home tonight and we can have a catch up. I'm going to cook your favourite dinner and I might even do a dessert."

"I'll look forward to that, Mum. I'd better go and get organised. Dad is going to drop me at school on his way to work." Lizzie said, getting up and heading to her bedroom.

I was thankful she'd been such an understanding and easygoing child. She had never caused us any grief or worry.

The house was soon quiet. I hung out the washing and did as much as I could before the first woman arrived. People might have thought that having a clinic at home would feel intrusive, but I always found it nice to be home.

The women coming today were all at various stages of their pregnancies. I had my notes sorted in order of their arrival and information sheets ready to give out according to their stage of pregnancy.

I took bloods from a couple of the women during the morning

and also had taken some swabs that I needed to drop off at the medical centre. I had a break early in the afternoon when I could go up town and drop them off.

I drove to the medical centre with the samples, planning on having a bite to eat and a coffee when I got back home. I rushed in and, as I opened the door, I was confronted by a stand of pamphlets. I don't know why they took my eye so instantly.

Stopping for a minute, I took one from the stand and opened it up. The pamphlets were advertising a midwifery practice in Palmerston North. I looked around and saw that the pamphlets I had left before I went on holiday were nowhere to be seen. Stunned, I dropped off the samples and got back into the car.

'What does this mean?' I thought as I started to drive away.

I knew that I seldom got referrals from the medical centre, but to support and promote midwives from Palmerston North seemed like a kick in the guts – the ultimate insult. After seven years of working as the independent midwife in our community, I thought that the barriers might have been broken down. Certainly, the women had embraced me. I felt very much appreciated by them and had endeavoured to give them the best care possible.

I went home and made myself a sandwich and a cup of coffee, pondering what I had just seen and why it had affected me so much. I was almost shaking with emotion, trying to bring reason to my mind and not be overcome.

This latest incident had affected my Achilles' heel – my weakness of feeling rejected. Thoughts whirled around in my head. 'Just get over it. You have the support from the women – what more do you want?' I said to myself.

I knew that no one was obliged to give me referrals at all. I should just toughen up and not let things worry me so much. Certainly, I wasn't a businesswoman, but I had never wanted or pretended to be. I was just a midwife wanting to give first class care to women who trusted me. I kept reassuring myself, reasoning what I was feeling and fighting the side of me that just wanted to burst into tears.

I still had three more appointments to go, so I mustered up the strength to carry on. I put all the negative thoughts out of my mind and gave the women my full attention.

After the last women had gone, the thoughts came back. I wondered why this had happened and what was wrong with me. My work was good and I had never had any adverse outcomes, which I was constantly thankful for.

I started thinking about dinner and what to cook. I looked at what was in the fridge and decided on lasagne with a salad and ginger steamed pudding – one of Lizzie's favourite dinners.

'That will go down a treat with both Barry and Lizzie,' I thought.

I wanted to make a bit of an effort since they had been fending for themselves over the past two weeks.

As dinner was cooking, I sat down and started looking through the mail that had come since I'd been away. I methodically opened all the uninteresting bills and other business-related mail. The Midwifery News was there and I started flicking through the pages, relaxing as I looked for some interesting reading. The articles were always interesting and it was good to keep up to date with what was happening in the midwifery world.

As I turned over the pages, an advertisement caught my eye. The advertisement was recruiting midwives to work in Cambridge in the United Kingdom. I studied the advertisement more closely. An agency was advertising on behalf of Addenbrookes Hospital, where they needed midwives, and the agency would help with visas and whatever was needed. There was a phone number to ring.

My heart leaped and I couldn't stop thinking about the possibility of working in England. I had thought about going to England for a trip, but working and living over there had never crossed my mind.

I couldn't wait for Barry to arrive home, so that I could talk to him about the possibility of living and working in England. Maybe a new chapter in our lives was opening up – and the world with it.

"Well, what do you think, Barry? Do you think I should enquire about working in England? I know it would take a lot of planning, but what an adventure. If we went and worked there, just think of what we could see and do. I have always wanted to travel, but we have never had the opportunity."

I was beside myself with excitement. I had hope in my spirit and something to plan for. A new stage in our lives was opening up. We thought and planned and thought again, going over how to make this developing dream happen and what the possibilities were.

From the time the agency was contacted, it seemed like dominos were falling in succession and the Red Sea was parting. In that year – the planning year – my sister and I went on a trip to England and I had my interview at Addenbrookes Hospital. I got a position starting at 'The Rosie' in the following February.

We put our house on the market as soon as I had confirmation of a position. In stark contrast to when we went to Wanganui and our house had no potential buyers, this time our prayers were answered

– the first people who viewed the house bought it. As we talked and planned, Barry and I decided that we couldn't move Elizabeth when she was so close to finishing school. It wouldn't have been fair on her to be uprooted when she was so close to her planning her life and what she wanted to do.

"I have to go in February," I said to Barry. "The door may close if we don't act now. They might not need any more midwives once they have recruited enough. This advertisement has probably gone worldwide."

"Honestly, I don't mind staying back and coming over the following year. You'll have your registration then and a place to stay rather than the hospital quarters," he said.

"That would be fantastic if you don't mind. I will be studying and doing the adaptation course in the first year anyway. Maybe you could come over during the year for a holiday to break up our time apart."

The planning took nearly a year, with all the practical hurdles we had to go through and requisite paper war. We took each step in our stride, working through the lists of things we needed to do.

From the time we made the decision to go to England, I stopped taking new bookings. I was able to look after all the women who had already come to me, since it took so long to get everything organised. My last birth was on Christmas Day 2003. It seemed fitting that my last birth as an independent midwife was on Christmas Day.

It was an exciting time and a new adventure into the unknown was beginning. A new chapter of our lives was opening up. Maybe there would be other countries in the world where my skills as a midwife would be needed. Barry was with me and that was the most important thing. He was by my side – not always physically, but he was there nevertheless.

I pondered life and the future. The journey of life continues and so, too, does my dream of helping to bring life into this world. I thought I had reached my dream when I became a midwife, but the dream has developed as the journey has continued. With every stage of life comes another adventure and, with it, its own challenges.

My passion is driven by Shelley, my baby who never made it – it is her that spurs me on. I dream that someday I will meet her and that thought brings tears to my eyes, still. I imagine her in my mind and dream of that moment.

Acknowledgements

THANK YOU TO MY HUSBAND Barry, my best friend and companion. You have been so faithful and loyal. Thank you for our journey and your listening ear. I love you.

To Rae McGregor, thank you for your guidance, advice and experience. Your help has been invaluable and this book would not have been completed without your encouragement and help.

Thank you to my family for their love and support. To my children who have grown up to be my best friends and to my grandchildren who make getting older so worth it.

A special thank you to Elizabeth for editing this book.

To my parents, Daphne and Ian Watts. Thank you Mum for teaching me so many skills that have helped me in life. Thank you Dad for showing me that peace is better than strife and that to love others is the most precious gift we can give.

Thank you to my Lord and Saviour Jesus Christ for giving me life and making life beautiful.

Printed in Great Britain
by Amazon

62738691R00167